Wines

For

Health

By

Joseph Bertuccio

The Wine Specialist

Since 1969

Wine Etiquette International
5 School Lane
Lloyd Harbor, New York 11743
631-271-1610
E-mail: Wineetiquette@aol.com

Printed by
CreateSpace

Printed in the United States of America
First Edition
1 2 3 4 5 6 7 8 9 10

EDITED   MARY LOU NICHOL

COVER DESIGN BY CORIN HIRSCH

DESIGNED BY ALEX NARTOWICZ

JOSEPH BERTUCCIO

WINE ETIQUETTE INTERNATIONAL

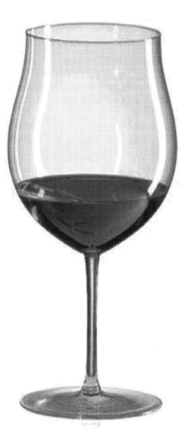

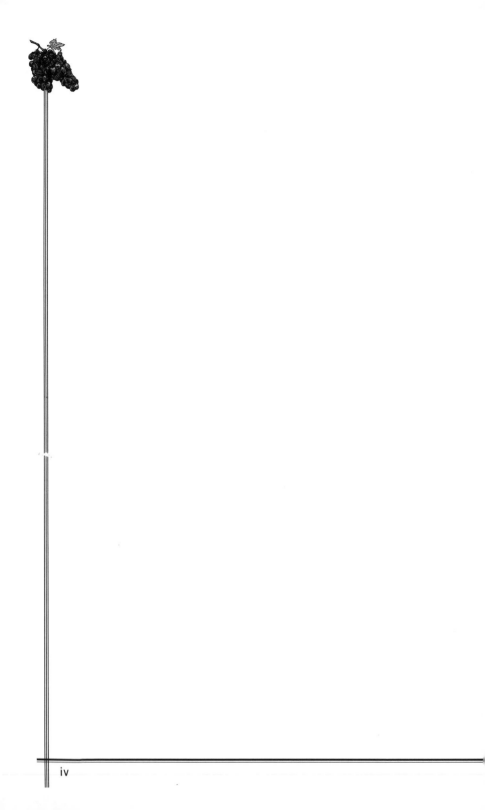

In Memory of

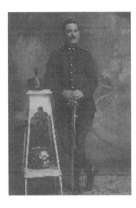

Lodovico Polizzotto
"My Grandfather"
"Cavaliere"
One of the Last Standing Soldiers
Battle of Monte Terzo 1914-1918
World War I

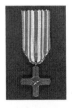

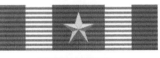

Nastrino della medaglia di cavaliere dell'Ordine di Vittorio Veneto.
English
Ribbon of the Italian Medal of Knight of the Order of Vittorio Venento

Contents

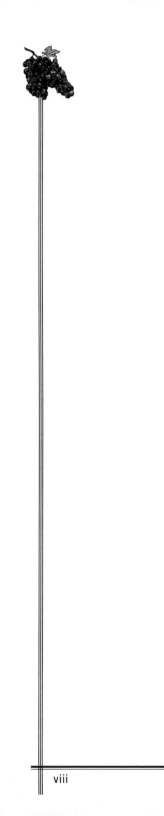

Disclaimer...

Maybe I should have dedicated this book to our forefathers who gave us constitutional permission to express ourselves through free speech in the United States.

As you read my book cover to cover, please note that I am not a medical doctor, witch doctor, wine doctor, astrologer, psychic, a member of any cult, etc.

Growing up, I was a Cub Scout, Boy Scout, Explorer, Civil Air Patrol member, and lieutenant cadet in a military academy. In my later years, I was a volunteer fireman, community Santa, and recent member of CERT (Community Emergency Response Team), a division of the United States Department of Homeland Security.

This book is for educational purposes only. All contents are my opinions and thoughts. I suggest you consult with your licensed medical doctor before taking any action regarding what you read in this book. Remember, you alone are responsible, not the author, publisher, distributors, bookstores, Internet stores, etc., if you choose any behavior based on what you read on the following pages.

This book is intended for readers over twenty-one years of age. Consuming alcoholic drinks should always be in moderation. I am in total support of MADD (Mothers against Drunk Driving) and SADD (Students Against Destructive Decisions).

Joseph Bertuccio

x

FORWARD:

People are living longer today than fifty years ago. Why? Well, you know most of the reasons and answers.

But there is one fine find in the universal search for the ingredients in the fountain of youth that is right under our noses, so to speak, and has been for years. That is wine and the benefits of wine for health. I'm talking about all the benefits wine offers your body.

Recent studies show that certain wines and spirits increase longevity as long as we drink in moderation.

Unlike previous studies, which included beer and alcohol, one recent study shows only wine is associated with longevity. Over thirteen thousand men and women ages thirty to seventy participated in a twelve-year Copenhagen Heart Study that revealed that those who drank wine daily were much less likely to die during the study period than those who drank beer or hard liquor or no alcohol at all. 1

I also look at it this way. In some circles, wine is labeled "the nectar of the gods," and who am I to criticize that? If wine and spirits (liquid spirits,) are mentioned in the Bible, then they're a good thing. So if they're a good thing, why shouldn't they help the human body? I'm sure I will get hundreds of letters to debate that wine and spirits are also bad. But that's not what this book is about.

In my forty years of experience in the wine industry, I have met many people who say they can't drink wine or spirits because they have an allergic reaction to them or because wine and spirits don't agree with their internal system. This may be true, but I have narrowed it down to about 1 percent of these people who are truly allergic in some way. Now, what about the other 99 percent?

They may have thought they were allergic, but after I recommended wine and spirit remedies, they are now drinking and cooking with wine. And no side effects!

I can honestly say that I have a wine for everyone's palate and pocketbook. In this book, you will surely appreciate the synergy between wine and spirits for health and, who knows, maybe someday they will save your life.

"Good wine is a good creature, if it be well used."
William Shakespeare, *Othello*

Chapter 1

GRAPE POWER

When I think of grapes, I cannot help saying to myself, "Ah, yes, the fruit of the vine."

Grapes come in all colors and sizes. We enjoy consuming grapes in all forms of juices and jellies. They're very tempting and delicious; I dare you to eat just one. Please eat grapes in moderation. Eat too many at one time and the juices could, as I would like to think, ferment and make you very uncomfortable. If you know what I mean!

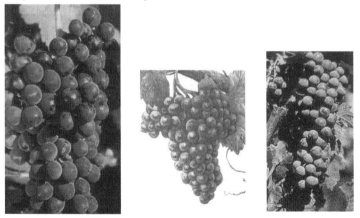

I heard a story once of a couple who started a small vineyard in Virginia. Yes, did you know Virginia has vineyards and wineries that produce exceptional varietals? Did you also know that Thomas Jefferson planted one of the first vineyards in the United States at his estate, Monticello, in Charlottesville? His long-lasting experiments with European vines gave him the unofficial title of America's "first distinguished viticulturist." He was also known as wine adviser to Presidents Washington, Madison, and Monroe.

I like to think I have a little of Thomas Jefferson's vision too, because I was asked to select dinner wines for President Gerald Ford when he was in office.

But enough of this wine trivia. Let's get back to my story.

A True Cork Tale

It was harvest time in beautiful Virginia. Fall was just around the corner. The grapes were ripe and full of juice. It was time to pick the grapes and declare a new vintage.

There was just one problem facing this young couple who owned the vineyard: they didn't have enough help to pick the grapes.

When a nearby vineyard heard about their dilemma, the owners offered their grape-picking machine. They borrowed the machine and were able to complete their harvest. This machine is quite large and is in the shape of the small letter n. It covers over the grape vines when driving through the rows in the vineyard.

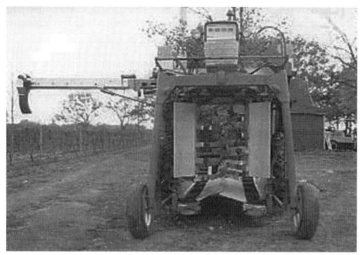

As the machine passes the vines, it agitates and shakes bunches of grapes onto a conveyor belt that allows the grapes to fall into a trailing hopper.

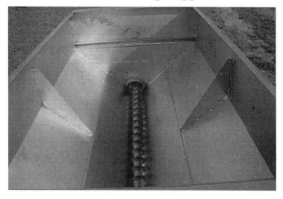

Although 99 percent of the grapes are not damaged by this technique, there are always some damaged grapes that are bruised and cut lying on the ground.

The day after picking all the grapes, the couple noticed hundreds of dead birds lying throughout the vineyard. They were shocked and didn't know what killed the birds. They immediately hired a few workers to gather the birds and bury them in a large hole dug by their backhoe.

When the workers began to gather the birds, they noticed the birds were alive and moving as they picked them up. It seems that the birds ate the damaged grapes and were inebriated from the lacerated grape skins that fermented.

Rumor has it that the following year, there were twice as many birds waiting for the machine to pass through the vineyard.

Can you remember drinking grape juice when you were a kid? Do you remember your mom saying, "Drink up all your juice, it's good for you"?

OK, maybe that was milk! But, if Mom had known about the benefits of the antioxidants and polyphenols in grapes then, as we do now, I bet we would have been drinking a lot more grape juice.

What about White Grape Juice?

The latest studies report white grape juice contains fewer antioxidant polyphenols than purple. What is a polyphenol? you ask. According to Dr. Harvey Finkel, a clinical professor of medicine at Boston University Medical Center and a frequent contributor to the AIM (Alcohol in Moderation) Quarterly Digest:

"The antioxidant polyphenol is not only found abundantly in red wine, it also plays a significant part in the production of the vine itself. It acts as a fungal protection and contributes to the color, flavor, and texture of the wine.

Polyphenol acts as an antioxidant that protects against bad tissue damage in the body and is also associated with cancer prevention."

On the subject of color, did you know that red and rosé wines get their color by the contact between red grape skins and the freshly pressed grape juice? Although all grape juice is clear when freshly pressed, the skins are what give the wine color. The longer you leave the red grape skins in contact with the fresh wine juice, the darker the wine will get. It is safe to say that you can make white wine from a red grape. I like to stump people with that one.

Wines for Health

Let's do some detective work.

If we know there's less polyphenol in clear white grape juice or clear white wine than there is in red wine, it makes sense the antioxidant polyphenol is in the tannin that is derived from grape skins in making wine and grape juice.

In wine making, tannin is also found in the seeds and stems, which are discarded before fermentation. Tannin is one of the most important constituents in red wine and plays a key role in the character, texture, quality, and flavor of the wine.

This does not mean that you should stop drinking white wine. On the contrary white wine is also good for other ailments of the body, which I discuss later in this chapter.

As some of the same grape varietals are grown in different and diverse wine regions all around the world, the wines made from those grapes will not have the same exact character, texture, quality, and flavor. Why? Because of the many variables that have to be taken into account.

Among them are the growing conditions of the different wine regions (terroir), which include the location of the vineyard, soil content, climate, and wine-making techniques. All these variables reflect heavily in the taste of the wine.

Have you ever compared a cabernet sauvignon (cab) from Chile with a cabernet sauvignon from Napa Valley, California? If you have, you will agree that the same grape varietal from South America will have a deeper purplish hue in the robe (the wine coating in a wine glass). If you swirl a glass of each, you will notice that the grape varietal from South America will have a more earthy texture resulting in a stronger aftertaste.

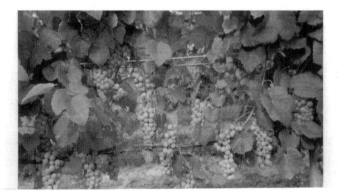

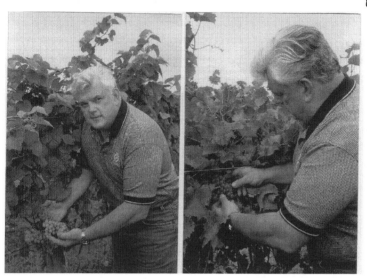

Where does this earthiness come from? It comes from the soil.

The vine absorbs the minerals from the soil and passes them through the stems and seeds and into the grape skins, giving a unique flavor to the grapes. Once the grapes are crushed, the tannins from the skins are released into the wine.

Now that we know red wines have more tannin than whites, how do we detect this when tasting? It's easy. When you taste a red wine, your mouth immediately reacts to a dry, bitter taste toward the back of your tongue. You will also detect a dry blotter feeling between your cheeks and your gums if there's a high amount of tannin.

Tannin does not ruin a red wine. It enhances the structure (firmness or softness), depending on how much tannin is present. Without tannin, a wine will not age properly. Yes, there are many factors in aging wine, but tannin is one of the basic elements.

Red Wine Every Day

Now that we have a good idea of why grapes have health power, let's delve a little more deeply into the varietals that have the most punch (no pun intended).

Grapes contain a natural bacterial ingredient called resveratrol that prevents human blood cells from becoming cancerous. Resveratrol is a free-radical-fighting antioxidant that penetrates existing malignant cells, making it impossible for them to spread. Keeping this in mind, a healthy diet of fruits, nuts, vegetables, and red wine, all consumed in moderation, could prevent you from getting cancer, or help prevent a cancer from spreading. Isn't this worth trying? What do you have to lose? It's all healthy intake for your body.

And there's more. Not only does wine contain resveratrol, but it also contains flavonoids from the grape skins, stems, and seeds. Flavonoids contain antioxidants that produce a better HDL–LDL (good-bad) cholesterol ratio.

Technically speaking, resveratrol is found in all red wine, and it helps fight against heart disease, dementia, and Alzheimer's disease!

It Gets Better!

The "French paradox," a term just about set in stone (1991), gave overwhelming evidence that drinking moderate amounts of red wine daily reduces the risk of heart attacks despite a high intake of saturated fat.

Dr. Serge Renaud, director of the French National Institute of Health and Medical Research, felt the paradox was due to the wine-drinking habit in France.

Many favorable studies pouring in from medical institutions all over the world concur that red wine has anti-aging properties and is good for the heart if taken regularly in moderate quantities.

Let me define the term *moderate quantities of wine*, according to the U.S. Department of Agriculture's "Dietary Guidelines for Americans." For women, no more than one drink a day (5 ounces), and for men, no more than two drinks a day (10 ounces). To be most effective, wine drinks should be consumed with a meal. This doesn't mean a cheeseburger and French fries.

Remember, the antioxidants break down in the grapes together with the polyphenol compounds in the wine. This process helps the body absorb the alcohol easier when drinking and eating moderately compared to the drinking of hard liquor.

Here is some international evidence to back up *Wines for Health.*

1993: Harvard School of Public Health developed a Mediterranean diet program that included wine as part of the recommended diet. In 1995, dietary guidelines for

Americans admitted for the first time that moderate drinking of wine might reduce the risk of coronary heart disease among males forty-five years of age and older and women sixty-five years of age and older.

1995: A study conducted in Copenhagen from 1976 to 1988 on over thirteen thousand men and women between thirty and seventy years of age concluded that those who drank between three and five glasses of wine a day had half the mortality risk of those who did not drink at all or drank beer and hard liquor drinks.[1]

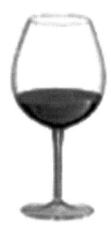

In a recent study by the American Cancer Society conducted on nearly five hundred thousand men and women. It concluded that a drink a day can, by middle age, cut the risk of premature death by 20 percent.[2]

New studies show the health benefits of alcohol. Recent reports published by the American Heart Association (AHA) and the *American Journal of Cardiology* are providing further support of the theory that moderate alcohol consumption cuts the risk of heart disease and stroke.

2000: Scientists at Northeastern Ohio University's College of Medicine and Pharmacy discovered resveratrol could also prevent the spread of herpes, and that this compound in red wine, when put on the open sores (including facial sores), can reduce them from growing fully.[3]

They also claimed that putting resveratrol in condoms and contraceptive foams can prevent the spread of genital herpes.

Move over, Airborne. Here comes red wine again, for the common cold.

Let's start a petition that all airlines serve a glass of red wine to all passengers over twenty-one years of age to help their immune systems and try to prevent colds from coming on.

Wine and Common-Cold Research Findings

In 2002, a team of doctors from the University of Santiago de Compostela, University Hospital of Canary Islands, and Dr. Miguel Harnan of Harvard School of Public Health in Boston studied 4,272 teachers in five universities for one year. All the males and females regularly logged common-cold conditions like sneezing, sore throat, running nose, cough, and headaches. The study indicated that people who drank a daily average of more than two glasses of wine experienced a 40 percent reduction in these conditions compared to those who did not drink any alcohol.[4]

Wine and Peptic Ulcers

A study published in January 2003 in the *American Journal of Gastroenterology* showed that moderate, regular drinking of wine or beer decreases the risk of peptic ulcers and may help rid the body of the bacteria suspected of causing them. Both over consumption, especially of beer, and any regular consumption of spirits at even a low level increased the risk.

Several European studies have shown that the prophylactic effects of regular to moderate alcohol consumption may include the prevention or postponement of Alzheimer's, Parkinson's, and other forms of dementia.

Compounds in resveratrol reduce the number of fat cells, and they may one day be used to treat or prevent obesity, according to a new study.

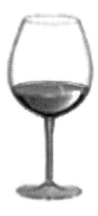

Researchers at the University of Ulm in Germany wanted to know if resveratrol could mimic the effects of calorie restriction in human fat cells by changing their size or function. In the cell-based study, they found that resveratrol inhibited the pre-fat cells from increasing and prevented them from converting into mature fat cells. Resveratrol also hindered fat storage. Most interesting, according to Pamela Fischer-Posovszky, PhD, a pediatric endocrinology research fellow in the university's Diabetes and Obesity Unit, was that resveratrol reduced production of certain cytokines, substances that may be linked to the development of obesity-related disorders, such as diabetes and clogged coronary arteries. Also, resveratrol stimulated formation of a protein known to decrease the risk of heart attack.

Men who are "moderate" drinkers—between five and ten drinks per week—have a lower risk for adult-onset diabetes than either abstainers or heavy drinkers, researchers report. "Men with a high alcohol intake may be able to reduce their risk of developing type 2 diabetes if they drink less," report

Dr. Ming Wei and colleagues at the Cooper Institute in Dallas, Texas.

As reported previously by Reuters Health, numerous studies have suggested that having a drink or two per day appears to have a protective effect against cardiovascular disease. In their study, Wei's team examined rates of type 2 diabetes—the adult-onset form of the disease affecting 95 percent of all diabetics—in over eighty-six hundred Texan men. They found that diabetes risks were lowest in men who drank between five and ten drinks per week, compared with either abstainers/infrequent drinkers (zero to five drinks per week) or heavy drinkers (ten to twenty-two drinks or above). In fact, infrequent or heavy drinkers faced twice the risk of type 2 diabetes of moderate drinkers!

Wei told Reuters Health that, according to previous studies, moderate drinking "reduces insulin resistance," while heavy alcohol consumption "increases insulin resistance." Insulin resistance—in which the body gradually stops responding to the sugar-hoarding effect of the hormone insulin—is thought to precede full-blown type 2 diabetes. Based on their findings, the authors estimate that "24 percent of the incident cases of diabetes in (adult men) might be attributable to high alcohol intake." While they do not recommend that abstainers take up drinking to lower their diabetes risk, they urge heavy drinkers to cut back in order to lower their risk.

Moderate drinkers may be less likely to develop blockages in the arteries that supply blood to the legs. In a study of almost four thousand people over fifty-five, Dutch researchers found that all women and nonsmoking men who reported having one or two drinks a day were less likely

than nondrinkers to have peripheral arterial disease (PAD).
These results complement previous research that suggests
light drinking can reduce cardiovascular disease risk.

The strongest effect was noted in nonsmoking women, who
were 59 percent less likely to have PAD than teetotalers.
PAD occurs when arteries in the legs become blocked by a
buildup of fatty material, a process known as atherosclerosis.
PAD can lead to leg cramps when walking. Atherosclerosis
in general can bring on stroke and heart attacks. Alcohol
may slow atherosclerosis by inhibiting the oxidation of
cholesterol, which prevents it from accumulating inside
arteries. Since atherosclerosis can lead to other
cardiovascular problems, reducing this process may be the
means by which light drinking promotes heart and blood
vessel health in general. The benefits of alcohol may stem
primarily from red wine. This could explain the stronger
effect seen in women, since women tended to choose wine,
whereas almost half of men liked beer best. 5

The new finding is consistent with the theory that the
resveratrol in red wine explains the French paradox, the
observation that French people eat a relatively high-fat diet
but have a low death rate from heart disease.

Other medical studies point to multiple benefits of regular,
moderate wine drinking that may include lowered risks of
stroke, colorectal tumors, skin and other types of cancers,
senile dementia. and even the common cold, as well as
reduction in the effects of scarring from radiation
treatments.

*"Researchers at University of Pittsburgh School of Medicine
reported that an antioxidant common to red wine and fruit might
help protect against radiation. Previous studies have shown that*

red wine can combat heart disease by reducing bad cholesterol and raising good cholesterol."[6]

Drinking Wine May Lower Risk for Upper Digestive Tract Cancer

Many studies have associated alcohol consumption with increased risk of upper digestive tract cancers. But Morton Gronbaek and colleagues at the Institute for Preventive Medicine in Copenhagen, Denmark, report just the opposite. They speculate that previous studies did not analyze data for specific types of beverages and/or did not distinguish between use and abuse. Although they acknowledge that their analysis may not be perfect, the Danish researchers tracked the thirteen-year incidence of mouth, throat, and esophageal cancers among twenty-eight thousand Danes. They report that heavy drinkers experienced a twelvefold increase in upper digestive cancers compared with abstainers. But among moderate drinkers, those who consumed at least 30 percent of their alcohol intake in the form of wine were at slightly lower risk than nondrinkers for these cancers. "A moderate intake of wine probably does not increase the risk of upper digestive tract cancer," the researchers concluded. They speculate that compounds found in wine, such as resveratrol, may exert powerful anticarcinogenic effects that protect against any cancer-causing effects of alcohol. "Wine contains several components with possible anticarcinogenic effects—these may exert their action locally in parallel with the possible effect of ethanol."

The nutritional contents of wine are minimal. There is no fat, cholesterol, or dietary fiber in any wine.

For Your Info

Here is the nutrition information for a single serving of wine, based upon a wine with a residual sugar content of 8 percent (a higher residual sugar increases the number of carbohydrates in the wine).

Type, Color: Dry red wine

Alcohol: 12.5 percent**
Single serving size: 6 ounces
Sodium: 8.5 milligrams
Calories: 123
Carbohydrates: 2.9 grams
Protein: 0.23 grams***

Type, Color: Dry white wine

Alcohol: 12.5 percent**
Single serving size: 6 ounces
Sodium: 8.5 milligrams
Calories: 115
Carbohydrates: 1.35 grams
Protein: 0.14 grams***

Type, Color: Sweet dessert wine

Alcohol: 18 percent**
Single serving size: 3 ounces
Sodium: 7.65 milligrams
Calories: 130
Carbohydrates: 10 grams
Protein: 0.17 grams***

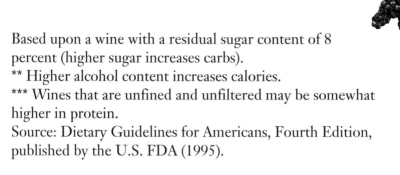

Based upon a wine with a residual sugar content of 8 percent (higher sugar increases carbs).
** Higher alcohol content increases calories.
*** Wines that are unfined and unfiltered may be somewhat higher in protein.
Source: Dietary Guidelines for Americans, Fourth Edition, published by the U.S. FDA (1995).

White Wine Health Remedies

Ok, maybe white wine has much less resveratrol and flavonoids than red wine because the skins and seeds are removed from the freshly pressed juices in production. But that's the only bad news.

The good news is that the regular drinking of red or white wine results
in 40% reduction of getting a cold. And for cigarette and cigar smokers here's more good news. White wine is good for the lungs.

A study by the University of Buffalo School of Medicine and Biomedical Sciences says that white-wine drinkers have healthier lungs than non-drinkers. These studies include red wine drinkers along with beer and spirit drinkers.

This study was headed by Dr. Holger Schunemann, Assistant Professor at the University of the American Thoracic Society. His team initiated the study to try to establish a link between wine drinking and lung health. The researchers studied a total of 1,555 residents of Erie and Niagara Counties in New York State who were 60 years old with no history of lung disorders.

Interviewers asked them about their dietary habits, smoking patterns, and alcohol consumption over the past thirty days and during their entire lives. Tests were completed on lung capacity and health. It was found that those who drank white wine only had the healthiest lungs—in terms of the breakdown of tissue with age, rather than specific diseases—followed by red wine drinkers.

Male wine drinkers may have a lower risk of lung cancer than those who drink beer or spirits. Dr. Eva Prescott and colleagues at Copenhagen University Hospital examined data from three Danish studies involving more than twenty-eight thousand adults. Overall, they found no association between low to moderate alcohol intake and lung cancer risk. When the analysis was limited to men, they observed that those who drank wine had a lower risk of lung cancer than those who did not drink wine. But the data also suggested an increased risk of lung cancer in men who drank beer or spirits. For example, men who reported drinking one to thirteen glasses of wine per week had a 22 percent lower risk of lung cancer compared with drinkers of other types of alcohol. Men who consumed more than thirteen glasses of wine per week had a 56 percent lower risk than other alcohol drinkers. The researchers suggest that the seemingly protective effect "may be related to the antioxidant properties of wine, and deserves further attention."

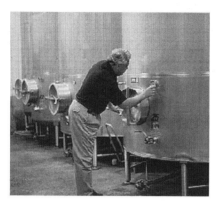

Here's a true story I would like to share with you...

I can remember, when I was seven years old, standing in front of then called Sloan-Kettering Hospital in New York City, waving up to my grandfather's window, because in 1957 children were not permitted to visit cancer patients. Yes, my grandfather was diagnosed with lung cancer because he smoked a gazillion cigarettes a day. I waved to him and he waved back before going into surgery to remove his right lung. I didn't clearly understand how severe that was, because I was annoyed that they wouldn't let me go up and see him.

After the operation, everyone in the family but me knew that doctors had given him two months to live. I remember him coming home to recuperate and drinking his little glass of white (moscato) wine with each meal every day. He also had an organic vegetable garden from which he ate everything he grew.

For the next twenty-five years, my grandfather got stronger and healthier. He outlived the doctors who gave him two months to live. During the twenty-five years, my grandfather was chauffeured to Sloan-Kettering once a month for a free checkup, and they recorded what he ate and drank.

With all the research I've been doing, I would like to think that it was good, healthy, organic food and white wine that kept him going for twenty-five years. But I would not rule out family, love, and divine intervention.

Consuming less than one alcoholic drink per day may help preserve the mental function of older women. Between 1995 and 1999, researchers interviewed 9,072 women, ages seventy to seventy-nine, in the Nurses' Health Study. Seven tests were administered to assess mental function. Information about the women's alcohol use had been collected at the beginning of the study in 1980 and was updated through 1994. After adjusting for other factors that could affect mental function, the researchers found that the women who drank moderately had better average scores on five of the seven tests and on a score that combined all seven tests. The effect seen on cognitive function was the equivalent of being one or two years younger.

Another Ongoing Study for White Wine

Could moderate consumption of white wine reduce the risk of arterial sclerosis occurring? Well, the jury is still out. But the most recent unofficial pilot studies taken over the last twenty years (Deutsche Wein Akademie) in Germany are

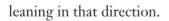

leaning in that direction.

Just ask Dr. Gustav Belz, PhD, FACC (Fellow of the American College of Cardiologists), professor of medicine at Johannes Gutenberg University of Mainz, Germany, and a senior physician at the Center for Cardiovascular Pharmacology, dealt with this problem. He concurs with suggestions resulting from an unofficial pilot study that data points to a finding that those who regularly drink moderate amounts of wine probably have less stiff, and therefore less sclerotic, blood vessels than comparable subjects who served as controls in the testing.

I also concur. You don't have to be a doctor of medicine to know that the risk factors for arterial sclerosis are high blood pressure, diabetes, stress, age, high blood fat rates, clogged and hard arteries, smoking, and inflammations. So if drinking wine in moderation helps fight against these risk factors, it's just a matter of time what the official studies will prove.

Would *you* like to wait for the results?

Here is some grape trivia…

Do you know where the world's oldest person lived?

Was it a man or a woman?

If you said "woman," you are correct. Her name was Jeanne L. Calment. The records show she lived in France, was 122 years old, and quit smoking two years before she died. She claims that her everyday diet included port wine and olive oil, among other foods. Oh, yes, I forgot to mention she was stress free and smiled every day.

CHAPTER 2

WINE - KNOW

As you learn more about the power of the grape, you should also learn about three wine categories:

still or table wine: 8 percent to 14 percent alcohol content

sparkling or effervescent: 8 percent to 14 percent alcohol content

fortified (strengthened with added alcohol): 17 percent to 22 percent alcohol content

All wine is living and breathing, whether in the bottle or in a barrel. I consider it as a live food and not a dead, processed food.

If you are familiar with bottles of red, white, or rosé wines, you will know they fall into the still or table wine category. For those bubbly people, and you know who you are, you're well familiar with the sparkling or effervescent wine bottles. You will find these bottles heavier because of the thicker glass used to support the extra pressure in the bottle.

Sparkling Wines

Effervescence distinguishes a sparkling wine from a still wine. Produced in different countries, sparkling wines are sometimes referred to by names particular to their country of origin. However, a sparkling wine by any other name is still a sparkling wine. All champagnes are sparkling wines, but not all sparkling wines are labeled "champagne." The reason goes as follows:

In Champagne, France, around the seventeenth century, a Benedictine monk by the name of Dom Perignon, the cellar master at the Abbey of Hautvillers, thought of a way to keep the sparkle in his wine. He contained the pressure with a stronger bottle and a thicker stopper, the forerunner of today's cork.

His improved techniques and creative cuveé (blending) gave new life to the "bubbly." Sparkling wines "arrived" in Champagne. This region is now known for the world's best sparklers, which are labeled for their district, Champagne (with a capital *C*), and referred to by that name. Today's law in France will not allow the word "champagne" on any sparkling wine, unless produced in the Champagne district.

Sparkling wines are also made outside this district of France by the champagne method; some can bear the name *methode champenoise*, others only *vin mousseux* (sparkling wine). These sparklers cannot carry "Champagne" on their label.

The *methode champenoise* process is laborious and expensive, and the resulting quality reflects the pride of the winemaker. Its success in producing a sparkling wine similar to Champagne has led other countries to imitate this method in the making of their own sparkling wines.

Spain has its *cava*, Germany has its *sekt*, Italy its *spumante*.

Some sparkling wines made in the United States, however, do bear the word "champagne" on their label. The reason for this is that during Prohibition, it was difficult to get Champagne from France, so the domestic wineries made their own for speakeasies in the 1920s.

As wineries became more sophisticated in the United States, through the years many held to the old agreement with France by labeling their best "bubbly" *methode champenoise*. This stands true for French-owned vineyards in California producing by the champagne method, but not using the name "champagne" on the label.

AUSTRALIA
Champagne
Champagne Method

FRANCE
Champagne
Methode Champenoise
Vin Mousseux

GERMANY
Sekt

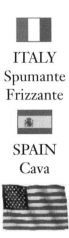

ITALY
Spumante
Frizzante

SPAIN
Cava

United States
Champagne

How Sweet It Is!

Most sparkling wines and all of the Champagnes from
France have their various degrees of sweetness printed on
the label.
Among the designations are:

brut—very, very, dry
extra dry—sweeter than brut, although dry
sec—medium sweet
demi-sec—quite sweet

Last but not least is the fortified wine category that can be
found in any size and shape bottle. Names for include
aperitif, digestivo, cordial, or an after-dinner drink.

Sherry

A still wine is fortified or strengthened with brandy in order to increase the alcohol content. These fortified wines are drunk as aperitifs, digestivos, or after-dinner cordials, or can be used in cooking.

The most popular fortified wines in the United States are Porto (port) from Portugal and sherry from Spain. With port, neutral grape brandy is added to the fermentation process to make a sweeter wine.

Sherry, on the other hand, is allowed to ferment much longer for the sugar to naturally change into carbon dioxide, producing a drier wine. Sherry brandy is added after fermentation.

Port Info

There are differences between the words "Port," "Porto," and "Oporto" when you see them on labels. Oporto is the city in Portugal from which the wine is shipped. Porto (original port wine) is the name of the imported wine. Port is a generic name found on bottles of that wine made in the United States and Australia. Although most ports are found to be red, white port is also produced. There are two types of Porto: vintage Porto and wood Porto.

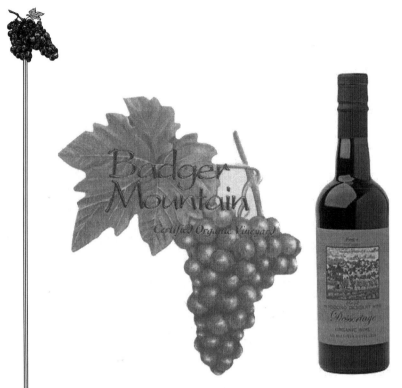

Vintage Porto

The wine produced in a year declared "vintage" by Porto producers becomes a vintage Porto. A vintage year creates the best possible conditions for the growing of grapes that particular year. Usually only one out of three years is declared a vintage year.

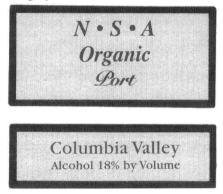

N • S • A
Organic
Port

Columbia Valley
Alcohol 18% by Volume

A vintage Porto matures in roughly ten to fifteen years, of which the first two years are spent in wood. This is usually a very small production of the best wine kept aside by the vineyard owner. Aging can only improve the quality of a vintage Porto in years to come. That is reflected in the price of a young vintage Porto at $45 and an older one from a prime vintage at over $100 a bottle.

Vintage Porto is considered a big, full wine, and it will develop a heavy crust with aging. This crust is made up of small particles that harden on the interior of the bottle.

It is very important that the wine is handled gently and decanted carefully. When decanting, you should let the clear wine pour off the crust, leaving it undisturbed, because it could break and cloud the wine.

Late Bottled Vintage Port

Vintage Ports that have been barrel aged four to six years before bottling have slowly lost their popularity among Port producers. Although they sound very stately and official, only a handful of Port shippers produce LBV Ports today. You will find these Ports labeled with a good vintage, and they are ready to be consumed as soon as they are bottled. There is no need to decant an LBV because the wine is filtered when bottled, which will reduce sediment with aging. And talking about aging, don't be fooled—LBVs cannot be compared to great vintage Ports, which continue to age much longer in the bottle.

Be aware when browsing in a wine shop for Ports that LBVs clearly show the vintage in large print, which can be misleading when reading the label and comparing prices to vintage Ports that usually cost 50 percent more.

Wood Porto

Tawny Porto is a blend of well-aged Portos of different vintages matured in oak casks. This wine is softer than both vintage and ruby Porto (below). It takes a long time to age and is very expensive.

Tawny Porto is pale in color because of all of its years in wood. From its original purple color, it turns to ruby red and then gradually to a golden-brown. Every time the wine is filtered to remove floating sediment, which is usually twice a year, the coloring matter also decreases.

Each producer of tawny Porto makes sure that the blend of taste that it acquires is always consistent for its label. Once bottled, it should be consumed early, for, unlike vintage Porto, it will not improve with age.

Ruby Porto is a blend of young wood Portos, usually from several different years. It is fruity and sweet with a bright ruby color. Like tawny Porto, it will not improve with age and it should be consumed early after bottling. Of all the Portos, ruby Porto is the least expensive. Both tawny Portos and ruby Portos are identified as such on the label.

Sherry

If you enjoy sipping sherry, then you will enjoy all the health benefits this fortified wine has to offer. Scientists from the University of Seville, Spain, claim that sherry could have the same effect on the body as red wine. A study shows that the polyphenols in red wine that are associated with preventing coronary artery disease are also found in sherry.

"Sherry is widely consumed, especially in Spain and the United Kingdom, and we have shown that its moderate intake decreased total cholesterol and increased HDL cholesterol," lead researcher Juan Guerrero said.

The *Journal of the Science of Food and Agriculture* shows that sherry reduces bad cholesterol and increases good cholesterol. Tests were performed on lab rats that were given a daily dosage of sherry equivalent to a 150-milliliter serving for a human adult. At the same time, other rats were given water or ethanol in water. A few months later, researchers found that the rats fed on sherry had less bad cholesterol and increased good HDL cholesterol, and that the sherry did not affect the weight of the rats or have any other significant impact on other metabolic processes.

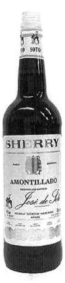

Scientists believe that polyphenols protect the heart's blood vessels by unclogging arteries that prevent bad cholesterol and lowering the potential of coronary heart disease.

Remember, these are preliminary test results and must be replicated by other researchers before they can be called fact. Here are some facts you should know when looking for a sherry to satisfy your palate. Sherries can be categorized as *fino* or *oloroso*.

FINO

A fino is created when nature continues the completed still-wine process and forms a white-colored film of yeast, called "flor," on the top layer of the wine. When flor develops, the wine becomes fino, producing a dry, distinctive taste.

The same process makes Manzanilla. It too is very dry and very pale, but has a lighter body than the medium-bodied fino. The grapes are grown and the wine is made in Sanlucar de Barrameda, Spain. Its microclimate of salt air and humidity is reflected in a slightly bitter hidden flavor in this sherry.

Amontillado is a dry, full-bodied, nutty fino with a pale straw to light golden color. It is usually a few degrees stronger in alcohol than fino. Amontillado is created when the flor doesn't make a white film and a darker film is present. This dark film is what gives the wine its nuttiness, a distinction in all Amontillados.

OLOROSO

Made from grapes that have been dried in the sun before fermentation, oloroso is a rich, full-bodied wine with a deep golden color, as compared to Amontillado. A true oloroso from Spain is dry, but there are sweeter olorosos produced named amarosos.

Cream sherries are produced from old olorosos, combining their golden color with a soft, cream style and full-bodied, sweet taste. They were developed and bottled in Bristol, England, from wine sent from Jerez, Spain. Over the years, cream sherries have become so popular worldwide that they are now also bottled in Jerez.

VERMOUTH

Have you ever heard the expression "Bitter to the tongue is sweet to the stomach"?

Vermouth producers claim this is true of their products. Some may say the Bible says to drink vermouth. Well, I won't disagree with them, but we know the Bible recommends you drink a little wine with every meal for good digestion. It could have meant vermouth. Why? Because enzymes, ferments, and organic acids in wine stimulate digestion.

Why is vermouth considered the most famous wine? Maybe it's because it is red wine steeped in the herb woodworm *(Artemisia absinthium)*. *Vinum absinthita*, known as its medicinal name, is made by soaking a handful of wormwood in a gallon of red wine for a little over a month in a well-sealed, stopped jar.

Ancient Greeks believed that absinthe wine was the antidote against the poison of mushrooms and hemlock. Over the years, vermouth was used for its medicinal powers to help expel intestinal worms and parasites. It calms an agitated, irritated, or hyperacidic stomach and is a cholagogue, meaning it stimulates the flow of bile. It is useful for many liver and gall bladder problems and restores the appetite. It reduces intermittent fevers, improves menstrual flow, hastens childbirth, and expels the afterbirth. It was also prescribed for jaundice, rheumatism, and anemia.

Other bitter tonic herbs that have been used in medicinal digestive wines and liqueurs include gentian *(Gentiana lutea)*, blessed thistle *(Carduus benedictus)*, chicory *(Chicorium intybus)*, dandelion root *(Taraxacum officinale)*, rhubarb root

(Rheum palmatum), and calamus root *(Acorus calamus)*. Because these herbs are quite bitter, their taste is improved with various sweet and/or pungent digestive tonics like fennel *(Foeniculum vulgare)*, licorice *(Glycyrrhiza glabra)*, cinnamon *(Cinnamomum zeylanicum)*, ginger *(Zingiber officinale)*, or cardamom (Eleteria cardamomum).

This wine-based product comes from countries all over the world. The most popular ones are from Italy, France, and the United States. They are made in many styles due to all of the different ingredients added by each company. Italy is known more for its sweet (red) vermouths and France for its dry (white) vermouths. Vermouth is used in mixed drinks such as the martini and manhattan. It is also used in cooking by many chefs throughout the world.

MARSALA

Marsala is known as Italy's cream sherry. It is produced in Sicily, where the volcanic soil is revealed in the unique-flavored undertones of a burnt, sweet sugar taste. This dark-colored dessert wine is used in the culinary world for dishes such as veal and chicken Marsala and in zabaglione, a world-favorite dessert.

MADEIRA

Named for the island from which it comes, Madeira is more popular for cooking than drinking. The two best known Madeiras found in the United States are malmsey or malvasia and rainwater. Malmsey is the sweetest of all Madeiras, dark brown in color and full-bodied. Rainwater is a blend of Verdelho, a sweet, soft wine; Bual, a sweet, golden dessert wine; and Sercial, the driest of all. All have an unusual "nose" and are excellent for enhancing the flavor of any meal.

Grape By-products

Here are some popular grape by-products (classified as brandy wine) available to help you fight what ails you.

Armagnac

Have you ever heard of Armagnac? If you're a brandy or cognac lover, I'm sure you have.

Armagnac is the oldest wine distillate of France. Originally, it was consumed for its therapeutic merits. In the fourteenth century, the benefits of Armagnac were written down, and in 1313, Prior Vital Dufor, a cardinal, claimed it had forty virtues. A translation stated: "It makes disappear redness and burning of the eyes, and stops them from tearing; it cures hepatitis, sober consumption adhering. It cures gout, cankers and fistula by ingestion, restores the paralysed member by massage and heals wounds of the skin by application. It enlivens the spirit, partaken in moderation, recalls the past to memory, renders men joyous, preserves youth, and retards senility. And when retained in the mouth, it loosens the tongue and emboldens the wit, if someone timid from time to time himself permits."

In the fourteenth century, we also find traces of its consumption and production. One can go back still further in time: Romans brought the wine-growing arts, the Arabs the distillation methods, and the Celts the barrel.

Between the fifteenth and the seventeenth centuries, more and more traces are found, and we can see that Armagnac is traded on the markets of Saint-Sever, Mont-de-Marsan, and Aire-sur-Adour. But Armagnac can thank the Dutch for its real commercial development.

Health benefits:

Research has suggested that Armagnac has health-enhancing qualities. Studies show that it can help prevent heart disease and serve to obviate obesity. Scientists at Bordeaux University have concluded that a moderate daily dose of Armagnac could lengthen one's life. For example, those living in Gascony, the area of France where Armagnac is made, tend to live around five years longer than the average in France. Some speculate that Armagnac's health benefits relate to its unique distillation process and aging. The southwestern area of France where Armagnac is produced has some of the lowest cardiovascular disease rates in the world. It has to be taken in moderation, though. The best amount seems to be three centiliters a day—greater amounts being potentially unhealthy. Researchers have concluded that Armagnac's health benefits are unrelated to its alcohol content. [7]

Armagnac (like cognac) is distilled from white wine grapes, namely the Folle Blanche, Ugni Blanc, and Colombard varieties. After distillation, it's aged in casks made primarily from local Monlezun black oak. The key technical difference between Armagnac and cognac is that the latter is distilled twice, whereas the former is distilled only once. This means more time in the oak for Armagnac; the extra patience required rewards us with a brandy with more finesse and roundness

VS on the label means the Armagnac has spent a minimum of two years in cask; VSOP and Reserve labels indicate five years; XO and Napoleon are aged six years; and Hors d' Age means ten years or more. The general rule when selecting a fine Armagnac is that the older Armagnacs are better, more complex, and more expensive, but it's also important to choose Armagnac from a good producer. When I first started in the wine and spirits industry, I was fortunate enough to represent and sell what I think is the finest Armagnac, Larressingle, in New York. I strongly recommend the Larressingle VSOP and XO bottlings, which are found in the finest wine shops.

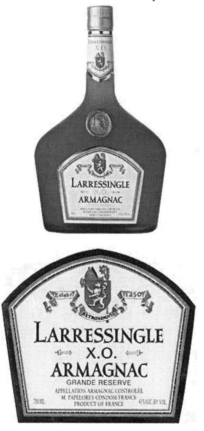

Brandy and Cognac

Brandy is made all over the world. It is a spirit made by distilling grapes to obtain a higher proof than ordinary still or table wine. Most brandy is made from grape wine. It can also be made from pomace, a mixture of stems and seeds left after the grapes have been pressed. Brandy can also be made from fermented juices other than grapes. The name is derived from the Dutch word *brandewein*, which means "fire wine."

You don't have to think twice when you take a shot of brandy. Monash University researcher Dr. Gordon Troup from the School of Physics said that, in moderation, brandy has been shown to have supplementary medicinal health benefits—and the better quality the brandy, the greater the benefit. The key to its benefit is antioxidants that come mainly from copper during the distilling process. He said a shot (thirty milliliters) of brandy would give the equivalent antioxidant potential to the daily recommended intake of vitamin C.

It stands to reason that the antioxidents in red wine are also found in brandy and that distillation does not play a role in removing them.

I'm sure you are familiar with all types of brandy. But did you know that brandy made in the Cognac region of France is called cognac and is produced under the strictest guidelines? The Cognac region stretches over two regions in western France, Charente-Maritime (bordering the Atlantic Ocean) and Charente (a little further inland). There are six crus (or growth areas) designated for producing cognac. Listed in descending order of aging potential and quality, they are as follows: Grand

Champagne, Petite Champagne, Borderies, Fins Bois, Bons Bois, and Bois Ordinaires.

Cognac, similar to Armagnac, grades its products based on their age counts.
VS (Very Special) or *** (three stars): aged at least two years in oak
VSOP (Very Special Old Pale): aged at least four years in oak
Napoleon or XO (Extra Old): aged at least six years in oak

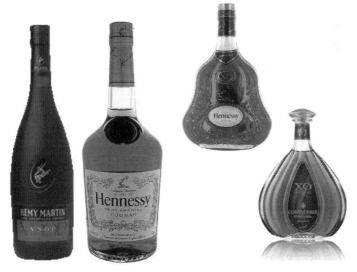

When buying a bottle of cognac, the general rule of thumb is that the older the cognac, the more money you will spend. This does not necessarily mean that it will taste better. As I always say, it depends on the individual palate. You may prefer a VSOP to a Napoleon.

Health Benefits: Although cognac is made from 100 percent white grapes, there is just as much data that support its benefits toward diabetes, cardiovascular disease, obesity, digestion, and some cancers as there is for wine from red grapes.

Cognac and Diabetes

Alcohol can have a negative effect on diabetics. Alcohol increases the "hypoglycemic" effect, which is found particularly in people suffering from diabetes, which increases the likelihood of comas. Many diabetics are advised to eat small and regular quantities of sugar to balance this effect.

One advantage of cognac is that cognac is very low in sugar content (0.32 grams, i.e., 128 calories, for a 1 1/2 oz. dose). This is very small when this is compared to the caloric value found in alcohol (91 calories) and this has proved important in the study of diabetes-obesity syndrome.

Studies have shown that moderate alcohol consumption has a favorable effect on the surrounding areas of insulin resistance and particularly on the adipocytes. Also, polyphenols contained in cognac have a vascular-protector effect due to the antioxidants' properties.

Cognac and Cardiovascular Disease

Indeed, alcohol in moderate doses has positive effects on the fat or grease buildup mechanisms and the formation of blood clots, limiting cardiovascular disease risks. The polyphenolic constituents assist in this effect of antioxidants and anticoagulants. However, keep in mind that alcohol consumption has to be controlled, even limited, in the case of obesity and high blood pressure. Cognac belongs to that sector of alcohol drinks that are rich in phenolic constituents with high antioxidant properties, as is red wine, and can contribute to reducing risks.

Cognac and Digestion

Ethanol has a double action on the digestive system but is very different from the action on cardiovascular problems. These possible effects on digestion lead to advice for moderate cognac consumption. However, the high quantity of polyphenols contained seems to play a role in adding to the protection effect of the gastric mucus membrane and is an extra protection factor.

Cognac and Obesity

It has been shown that a moderate consumption of cognac has no significant effect on men's weight and even has a mild slimming effect on women. On the other hand, individuals with hepatic and liver-related problems and risks should avoid drinking cognac.

Cognac and Cancer

Though alcohol, if moderately consumed, protects the cardiovascular system from disease and aids the digestion process, it can increase the risks of cancer of the upper aerodigestive tract. Cognac is rich in polyphenic constituents, and it has been shown in tests that the ellagic acid can inhibit cancer of the lung, liver, and esophagus.[8]

Grappa

As cognac is made in France using designated fine grapes, the same process in Italy would be used to make a wine called grappa, usually named after the varietal grape—for example, grappa de chardonnay. Grappa can taste harsh or smooth depending on the style of distillation. If you have ever had a bad experience tasting grappa for the first time, I bet it was distilled from pomace of inferior quality distillation and not the actual grape. This process is called grappa di Monovitigno, created by Benito and Giannola Nonino in December 1973. Monovitigno is a grappa of a single grape variety, such as moscato, Riesling, gewürztraminer, or picolit. The success of this distillation was so great that the Italian and foreign distillers followed this model, because this style of distillation produces a more superior grappa, reflecting a slight aroma and flavor of the original grapes.

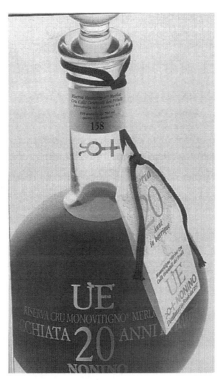

If you are thinking of trying grappa, I suggest you begin with Nonino and their many distillates available to choose from. After all, the Nonino family has been making grappa since 1897 when Orazio Nonino, the forefather of the family, founded his own distillery in Ronchi di Percoto, Italy. Until then, the distillery had existed only as a mobile still on wheels.

Today you will find the distillery is run by Beneto Nonino, his lovely wife, Giannola, and their three beautiful daughters, Antonella, Cristina, and Elizabetta.

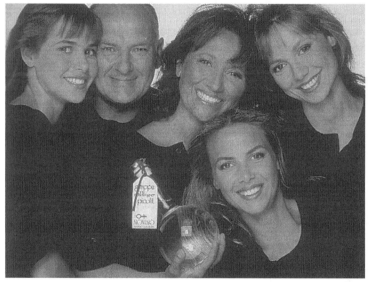

I had the pleasure of meeting the family while on a gastronomy tour by GRI (Gruppo Ristoranti Italiani) and the Friuli Venezia Giulia Tourism Board throughout Udine, Italy, accompanied by food writers.

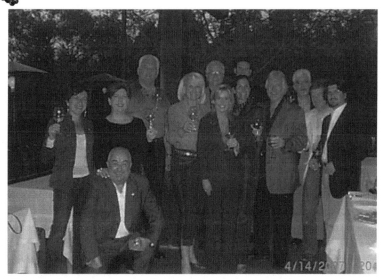

GRI and its many members support true, authentic Italian restaurants, pairing their menus with the traditional dishes and vino from that particular region. If you have never experienced this true cuisine from region to region, I suggest the next time you dine out, make sure the restaurant is a member of GRI for the best culinary experience from Italy.

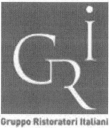

Gruppo Ristoratori Italiani
LEADING ITALIAN
RESTAURANTS IN AMERICA

It was in 1973 that Beneto and Giannola revolutionized the method of producing, introducing, and packaging Grappa in Italy and around the world. Nonino is credited with setting a trend of perfection in quality and style not only with the Italian government, but also with aristocratic palates in the finest wine circles.

If you have the opportunity to visit Nonino Distillery in Ronchi de Percoto, you will find the Noninos have re-established their artisanal batch steam still for the production of the Nonino distillates (grappas, honey, or fruit). They respect the tradition and the art of true craftsmanship.

You don't have to worry about the quality of the products they use, because the Nonino family personally oversees the purchase of the primary products and follows the various phases of distillation to guarantee the maximum quality of the distillate.

The Nonino family has five artisinal distilleries, each one with twelve batch steam stills for their production of unique distillates.

It doesn't matter which one of their five distilleries you walk through; when entering, you will get the feeling you are back in time. You will witness the stills in operation twenty-four hours a day, with slow, steady steam rising from the handcrafted still, capturing the true essence and flavor of the grapes, pomace to be converted to grappa. When standing among the steam stills, try closing your eyes and taking a deep breath to capture the unique aromas.

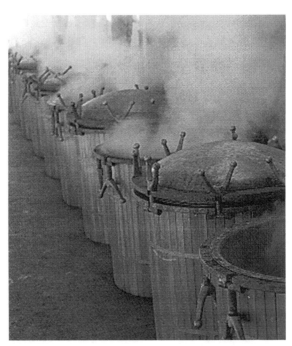

Remember any unique aroma you capture; you will again capture it tenfold when you sniff the finished product. Now, open your eyes and look around. You can't help but sense a mystical feeling come over you, like something out of a medieval scene.

I could go on and on and talk about how Nonino grappa uses the finest oaks, wild cherry, and pear in their barrels for aging their selection of distillates. But I have to get back to the finished products of Nonino and how they benefit the human body.

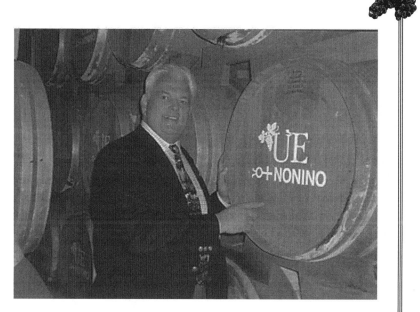

Whenever the Italians have a drink in their hands and are among people, they always make a gesture by holding the glass high in the air before drinking, saying "salute," a toast to good health. And why not? If you're drinking Nonino grappa, you can be assured it has more health elements from the grape pomace of a single varietal. The grape bunches are destalked and put into a temperature-controlled (stainless steel tanks) and an anaerobic-controlled environment upon arrival at the distillery to capture a rich bouquet in the finished product. This is unlike the process at most brandy distilleries.

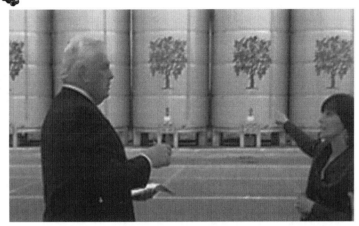

Grappa is the true brandy of Italy and it contains all the health benefits due to the selective grape control and distillation techniques.

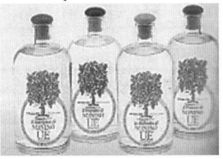

You can enjoy grappa straight, cook with it, or sip a caffé corretto (espresso corretto), a short cup of espresso with a shot of grappa.

Whether you drink Armagnac, brandy, cognac, or grappa, you now know they all play an important role in health benefits for the human body.

As a child growing up, I remember my grandpa always having a little glass of grappa (brandy) for what ailed him. A chest cold, a bad cough, a stomach problem, or just a

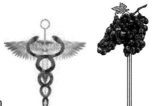

toothache—it seemed to do the trick.

How many of us know people like him? I'm sure you do, and I would love to hear your stories and remedies as well. Write to me. Who knows? Maybe I can use them in my next book.

Ready for a little detective work again? We know that alcohol kills germs, right?

We also know brandy contains at least 40 percent alcohol by volume and is made from the by-product of grapes (live food). Then it is safe to say that any distillate of grapes (such as brandy) mixed with any type of natural fruits, such as berries, apricots, plums, etc., can be good for the human body.

Wow! Do you see the pattern we are forming? Here are the pieces:

Grape antioxidants
Germ-killing alcohol
Healthy live food
Vitamin C from added fruits

All the right ingredients for what ails you. Case solved!

The next time you visit your favorite wine and spirits shop, take the time to look at all the different types of brandies on the market. You'll be very surprised. If you have some extra time, check out international fortified wines.

Read the labels; you might find a traditional fortified product of a particular country that not only has brandy as the base, but added herbs and spices to make up the traditional drink of that region. If it's a traditional drink, I bet it was used for medical ailments somehow.

Good hunting!

Ailment Tip

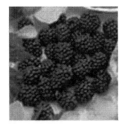 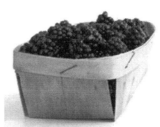

Here's a tip I've been using for years, and it works. The next time you have an upset stomach or you get diarrhea (I hate that word), take a couple of shots of blackberry brandy straight up. You will feel back to normal in about twenty minutes. You must use blackberry brandy (80 proof) and not blackberry liqueur (40 proof) with added sugar.

Fact: the American Indians used blackberries as medicine to cure stomach pain, heart disease, high blood pressure, and diabetes. Makes sense, doesn't it? Or does it? How did early Indians know about heart disease, high blood pressure, and diabetes? I guess they had a witch doctor!

Chapter 3

WINE RESEARCH

The scientific data just keeps pouring in from around the world. You can't believe how excited and happy I am to bring my readers all this positive news on how healthy the moderate consumption of red and white wine is. I feel like an archeologist who just uncovered a rare find. And what a find this is!

Here is what a BBC News article from Italy, titled "Health: A daily dose of wine could improve the brain," had to say:

"A glass and a half of wine a day could help improve the little gray cells and stop the progression of brain disorders, according to new research.

"Scientists at the Human Institute at the University of Milan say a chemical produced by wine could help a brain enzyme to function by up to sevenfold.

"According to the *New Scientist*, Alberto Bertelli and his colleagues have found that a chemical, resveratrol, found in grapes and wine, which fights infection in vines, helps the enzyme Map-kinase to regenerate neural cells.

"They tested the chemical on human neural cells in laboratory conditions and found it made them grow extensions, which helped them to connect up with each other."

Giulio Pasinetti, PhD, of Mount Sinai School of Medicine, and colleagues discovered the importance of grape seed extract to combat the incurable Alzheimer's disease (AD). They discovered the extract prevents amyloid beta in cells that forms toxic plaques that interfere with normal brain function.

Mice with symptoms of AD were exposed to the extract Mega Natural AZ for five months. They were given a daily dose of polyphenolic extract equal to polyphenols consumed by a person on a daily basis.

"After the five-month period, Alzheimer's mice were at an age at which they normally develop signs of disease. However, the extract exposure reduced amyloid beta accumulation and plaque formation in brains of Alzheimer's mice and also reduced cognitive decline: compared to placebo, extract-exposed Alzheimer's mice showed improved spatial memory. These data suggest that before symptoms begin, the grape seed extract may prevent or postpone plaque formation and slow cognitive deterioration associated with Alzheimer's disease." [9]

From Switzerland

Psychiatric Clinic, University of Basel, Basel, Switzerland, 2003:

> During the course of Alzheimer's Disease (AD), a neurotoxic substance called Amyloid peptide A - has been implicated to a great degree in cell death. Resveratrol, a natural polyphenol mainly found in red wine, has been shown to be cardioprotective

(heart) and chemoprotective (cancer). Since a moderate wine intake correlates with a lower risk for AD, an additional neuroprotective effect has been postulated for resveratrol.

Objective: The present study aimed at elucidating the possible neuroprotective effects of resveratrol against A -induced neurotoxicity.
Methods: The neuroprotective capacity against A -related oxidative stress was studied in a cell culture model suitable for studying such potentially neuroprotective substances.

Results: Resveratrol maintains cell viability and exerts an anti-oxidative action by enhancing the intracellular free-radical scavenger glutathione.

Conclusion: Our findings suggest that red wine may be neuroprotective through the actions of resveratrol.

"A new study from Harvard University researcher Gary Curhan and colleagues, using more than 81,000 women participants drawn from the Nurses' Health Study, found that an increase in fluid intake significantly reduces risk for kidney stones and that risk reduction was greatest for wine compared with other beverages. Out of seventeen beverages, including tea, coffee, fruit juices, milk, and water, wine was associated with the highest reduction in risk—59 percent." [10]

Also, researchers noted: "Intakes of caffeinated and decaffeinated coffee, tea, and wine were associated with decreased risk." Curhan and colleagues reported similar results for men and kidney stones in 1996. Wine consumption was associated with highest risk reduction—39 percent.

"There is evidence that moderate wine drinkers are less likely to develop dementia than heavy or nondrinkers. A study in the United States of America in 1998 shows that moderate wine drinkers have their visual cells preserved 20 percent better than beer or non-drinkers." [11]

"A small glass of wine will reduce tension, relax both mind and body, and aid digestion. Too much will cause drowsiness, impair judgment, and may lead to aggression. Clearly, moderation is needed, but there is no doubt that drinking wine can be beneficial. California researchers have shown that flavonoid components in grapes and wines inhibit the oxidation of low density lipoprotein by free radicals, which in turn has been related to several pathologies including that of ageing." [12]

Also, "Men who unwind after work with a glass of wine may be less likely to develop type 2 diabetes." [13]

Could wine become the new American drink?

A Gallup Poll in 2005 showed for the first time that Americans preferred wine over beer.

Is it possible that Americans are becoming more health conscious, or would you say they are acquiring a more sophisticated palate? I would like to think that it's a little bit of both.

If you asked my Sicilian grandfather who came from, in his words, the other side (meaning Palermo, Sicily, not the world beyond), a glass of wine was drunk every day with lunch and dinner. Even children were poured a little wine diluted with club soda or some type of frizzante (tiny spritz of bubbles). The grape was good for you. If you grew up in an Italian household, you know what I'm talking about.

Now don't write to me saying that children shouldn't drink alcoholic products. I don't condone minors drinking. I'm just saying this was done years ago on the other side.

At that time, the wine was pure and fresh, no additives. Grapes were grown in vineyards organically for families' own consumption. Many Europeans drank wine like the Americans drink soda pop, and who knows, maybe one day a Gallup Poll in America will show a preference for wine over soft drinks. Maybe it would cure obesity in young adults.

Whether that ever happens or not, it is a fact that wine consumption has nearly doubled in the past ten years, while beer consumption has grown less than 1 percent in the past eight years.

Chapter 4

Resveratrol for What Ails You?

Do you realize as every day passes more and more medical scientists and researchers are discovering the new benefits to the human body of moderate drinking of red wine that contains resveratrol?

As I was just finishing this book, I called a very good friend of mine, Dr. Robert Nuelander, an obstetrician-gynecologist who one of these days will host a *Wino-Gyno* television show with me. We have been kidding around with this concept for years, and now we have all the scientific and medical evidence to prove what we've been telling people for years.

I asked Bob if he would like to add a few paragraphs to my book, and, as a good friend, he was just as excited as I am to tell people about resveratrol.

Dr. Neulander writes:

The remarkable properties of resveratrol have been of tremendous interest, and researchers are trying to identify specific target proteins that allow for identification of enzymes that both are inhibited and activated by resveratrol.

Resveratrol is one of the numerous polyphenolic compounds found in vegetable sources. In recent years, the interest in this molecule has increased the potential major findings that have been shown to be used in cancer preventative measures and for heart protection as well as the positive effects on certain aspects of metabolism to increase lifespan and decrease Alzheimer's. The researchers have shown that anti-aging processes of resveratrol are quite evident.

The agent also has promising effects as an antioxidant, preoxidant agent, and it has also been used to enhance chemotherapy as well as in use of conventional chemotherapeutic agents to enhance their activities.

Numerous articles have been published. The connection that is of great interest is related to the diet and cancer of the Mediterranean countries. An article published in 2006 has an analysis of Mediterranean diet in relationship to common cancers in Italy. The high levels of resveratrol in their food certainly indicate that the digestive tracts have a decrease in cancer, and the risk of cancer with high levels of intake of vegetables and fruit certainly seeming to be directly correlated with this entity. It was concluded in Italy that adherence to the Mediterranean diet is a favorable indicator of decrease of several common epithelial cancers which are present. This was published in a Public Health Nutrition article dated December 2006. Other areas affected besides the digestive tract were the liver and kidney, which also showed very high levels of resveratrol.

In a review article in *Brain Research Review*, September 2006, resveratrol, which is a red wine polyphenol, was studied, and its effects were quite evident as protective measures against cardiovascular disease as well as cancer.

In another review article in *Nature Review* in June 2006, a study again showed resveratrol to be protective for the heart. It had other preventative measures as well, such as being a preventative agent for skin cancer and Alzheimer's, and it diminished aging. High levels of resveratrol also seemed to reduce stress and disease.

Importantly, resveratrol was reported to slow aging and increase lifespan in animal studies, as numerous articles focused. This was published most recently in *Current*

Medical Chemistry in 2006. Resveratrol has been shown to be very effective in numerous female cancers, such as breast cancers, specifically, as well as playing a very significant role in the inhibition of estrogen synthesis. As such, it is highly associated with diminished endometrial cancer effects, decreased pulmonary disease, decreased neurological disease, diabetes, and autoimmune disease, and exhibits a dysregulation of muliple cells signaling pathways that decrease inflammation. As far as hematologically, resveratrol has had effects on anti-platelet and blood clotting aspects.

It is very easy to conclude that resveratrol is a phenolic compound found naturally in fruits, nuts, flowers, wine (specifically red wine), seeds, and the bark of different plants.

Resveratrol as an integral part of human diet exhibits a wide range of biological effects including anti-cancer effects, anti-inflammatory effects, anti-cardiovascular aspects, anti-fungal properties, as well as anti-oxidant effecting agents, which go to Alzheimer's specifically.

In trying to analyze what resveratrol has and how it prevents cancer and other health problems, research has come up with a few answers. Resveratrol is a type of polyphenol called phyto-aloxin, a class of compounds produced as a plant's defense system against disease. It is produced in plants in response to invading fungal diseases, stress, injury, infection, and ultraviolet irradiation. Resveratrol is present in high levels in grapes and is found obviously in red wine, raspberries, peanuts, and plant compounds.

Red wine studies have found effects in several areas of cancers, including leukemia, skin, breast cancer, and endometrial cancers. Scientists are studying resveratrol to learn more about its anticancer prevention. Recent evidence in animal studies shows that the compounds may have a chemotherapeutic effect in the three stages of cancer. Drinking a glass of wine a day may cut in half a man's risk of prostate cancer, and the protective effect appears to be strongest against most aggressive forms of that disease. It also has been shown that men who consume four or more glasses of wine per week have a 60 percent lower incidence of the more aggressive types of prostate cancer.

It seems to me that research should continue in regard to the most effective role of resveratrol in anticancer prevention as well as in enhancing health and well-being. This is being studied in foreign countries somewhat more in depth than in America; however, a number of disease processes have been shown to be reduced by the specific properties of resveratrol.

The future has only begun based on all this information. There is an explosion of scientific information, as well as the pharmaceutical companies, such as GlaxoSmithKline, having tremendous interest in concentrating this and selling it in a tablet form of resveratrol; one is made by Sirtris Pharmaceuticals to help against multiple illnesses.

In the June 2008 *Wine Spectator*, "Science Tries to Harness Red-Wine Compound's Power," by Jacob Gaffney, says the scientific community is investing significant amounts of money to research the potential benefits of resveratrol. Two separate teams of researchers believe that the compound may have the ability to treat cells associated with disease. Gaffney goes on to say that one of the world's largest pharmaceutical firms, GlaxoSmithKline, announced that it would spend $720 million to purchase a smaller firm that has developed a synthetic form of this compound. And here's where I get very excited!

"Previous studies have shown that resveratrol bolsters healthy cells by stimulating mitochondria, organelles that provide energy for cellular operation. A new study suggests that resveratrol may enhance the efficacy of chemotherapy treatments."

The study was conducted at the University of Rochester and published in the March issue of *Advances in Experimental Medicine and Biology.*

"The team, led by Paul Okunieffm, MD, chief of radiation oncology at the university's cancer center, prepared two sets of pancreatic cancer cells and added pure resveratrol to one. After subjecting both sets to chemotherapy, they found that the resveratrol had shut down 35 percent of the mitochondria, thus allowing the cells to better receive the treatment." Is this priceless or what?

As I have been saying all along, resveratrol could someday be the key to help the human body fight against cancer.

"We already know about the heart-healthy effects of red wine, but new studies at Harvard Medical School and the Institute of Genetics and Molecular Biology have found that resveratrol may radically reduce the risk not only of heart disease, but of age-related illnesses such as Alzheimer's disease and dementia." [14]

"The Food and Drug Administration has already designated a lab-produced form of resveratrol (SRT501), made by Sirtris Pharmaceuticals, to help fight against an illness called MELAS— mitochondrial myopathy, encephalopathy, lactic acidosis, stroke-like episodes. MELAS is caused by mutated mitochondria and is a progressive and fatal disease that normally surfaces in patients between five and fifteen years old." Wine Spectator April 2008

Chapter 5

Why Pinot Noir?

If you're one of the millions who saw the Hollywood movie *Sideways* and switched from drinking merlot to pinot noir, you will be glad you did. Pinot noirs contain more resveratrol than any other red grape varietal.

The pinot noir grape is very fragile and hard to grow. It is said that the resveratrol bacterial fungi in the grape skins protect the grape in cool and damp climates. You will find this varietal grown in the Champagne and Burgundy regions of France, where it is of the utmost importance in the production of Champagne and red Burgundy wines. It is also grown in Australia, Canada, New Zealand, South Africa, Argentina, Brazil, Chile, Hungary, Italy, and the United States in California, New York (including Long Island), Oregon, and Washington.

Troy Creasy, Cornell University professor of fruit and vegetable science, recently completed an analysis of more than one hundred red wines from five states and foreign countries.

"Resveratrol concentration is measured in units called micromolar (μM), and an average red wine could have 3 to 4 μM. Wines above 5 μM of resveratrol are considered high; those above 7 are considered very high, and any product above 10 is extraordinary, Creasy said. New York wines used for this study came from Long Island, the Hudson Valley, the Finger Lakes, and the Lake Erie regions. The California wines came from the Central Coast, Mendocino, North Coast, and Sonoma. And the other U.S. wines came from Mississippi, Oregon, and the state of Washington.

Countries represented include Argentina, Australia, Canada, Chile, France, Italy, Slovenia, and South Africa. The average resveratrol content of all New York wines tested was 7.5 µM, compared with 5.8 µM for non-New York reds and 5 µM for California red wines. The type of wine with by far the highest resveratrol levels was pinot noir, with eleven of the seventeen New York wines registering above 10 µM. For pinot noir, the average levels were 13.6 µM for New York, 11 µM for all non-New York, and 10.1 µM for California."[15]

ICELAND

In 2006 AARP (the American Association of Retired Persons) magazine had an article written by Nissa Simon, a health writer, titled "The Power of Pinot Noir." The article states: "Red wine may reduce the risk of developing cataracts, according to the Reykjavik (Iceland) Eye Study. Among the 832 participants, those who drank moderate amounts of red wine (from two glasses per month to two or three glasses per day) had about half the risk of developing cataracts as nondrinkers, beer drinkers, and heavy drinkers. White wine was not included in the analysis. The findings were reported last year at a meeting of the Association for Research in Vision and Ophthalmology."

Can wine be humankind's oldest medicine? Well, there's an old Roman saying,
"In vino sanitas," which translates, "In wine there is health."

I can't think of any other older, natural fruit drink that can help so many parts of the human body.

How do you find a Pinot Noir to suit your budget? If you're

not familiar with the taste of this Burgundian-style wine, I suggest you start with a medium-priced PN (pinot noir) first. Why? Because if you start out buying the cheapest PN and don't like it, you will be turned off and probably go back to whatever you were drinking before you read my book. I don't want you to begin with a very good PN, because it might not fit into your budget if you were to drink a few glasses every day. Not everyone's palate is the same. You know the old saying, "Different strokes for different folks."

In the beginning of this chapter, I listed countries and states that produce PN wines. I suggest you visit your favorite wine shop and select a few different ones to taste. Trial and error puts you on the right track for a PN to satisfy your taste buds. Note: All varietals grown in different wine regions throughout the world will taste different. The synergy of soil and terroir play a very important part in how the wine will taste.

In France's Burgundy wine region (Cote d'Or), pinot noir is the predominant grape varietal. You will find the cost of these wines slightly higher than the norm, with the premier crus and grand crus more expensive. There are great PN bargains around if you know where to look. Try red wines produced a few miles south of the Cote d'Or in an area called Cote Chalonnaise. Made up of five main villages— Mercurey, Bouzeron, Rully, Givry, and Montagny—these areas produce less-expensive red wines. Reds from Givry and Mercurey especially can be sleepers when looking for quality and value.

Great pinot noir Burgundies include Aloxe-Corton, Bonnes Mares, Chambolle - Musigny, Clos de Vougeot, Gevrey

Chambertin, Grands Echezeaux, La Tache, Pommard, Nuits-St.-Georges, Richebourg, Romanee-Conti, and Vosne-Romanee.

Did you know that the most prestigious Champagne house, Moet, producing Dom Perignon, makes that wine with a PN varietal? And, if you're lucky enough to taste a rosé Champagne, you can be sure it will have some pinot noir blended into it.

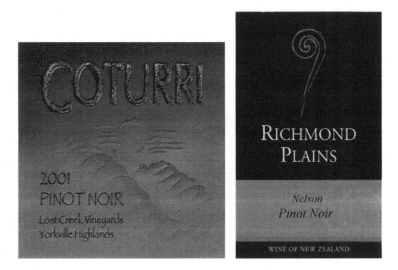

PINOT NOIRS TO LOOK FOR:

Jos. Drouhin Givry (France)
Jos. Drouhin Mercurey (France)
Jadot Pinot Noir 2006 (France)
Domaine Carneros Pinot Noir (Napa, California)
Foley Rancho Santa Rosa Pinot Noir (Lompoc, California)
Lincourt Pinot Noir (Santa Barbara County, California)
Benziger Signaterra Bella Luna Pinot Noir (Glen Ellen)
Tibor Gal Pinot Noir (Hungary)
Craggy Range Pinot Noir Te Muna Road (Hawkes Bay,

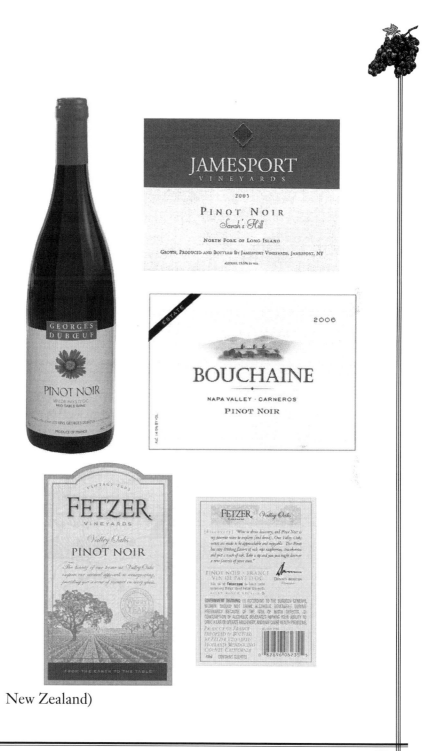

New Zealand)

Wild Rock Cupid's Arrow Pinot Noir (New Zealand)
Bouchaine Vineyards Pinot Noir (Napa, California)
Montes Winery Pinot Noir (Chile)
George Duboeuf Pinot Noir (France)
Guy Chaumont Borgogne Pinot Noir (France)
Richmond Plains Nelson Pinot Noir (New Zealand)

If you would like to try some award-winning pinot noirs
from Long Island, New York, you can choose from these:
Castello Di Borghese Pinot Noir Reserve (Cutchogue)
Castello Di Borghese Pinot Noir (Cutchogue)
Duck Walk Pinot Noir (Southampton)
Jamesport Vineyards Pinot Noir (Jamesport)
Martha Clara Vineyards Pinot Noir (Riverhead)
Osprey's Dominion Pinot Noir (Peconic)
Wolffer Estate Pinot Noir (Sagaponack)

Let's make a short list of what are now considered benefits
of moderate wine consumption.

- Prevents or reduces the effects of diseases such as cancer,
  heart disease, dementia, and Alzheimer's

- Improves HDL–LDL (good-bad) cholesterol ratio

- Reduces human mortality rate up to 30 percent

- Curtails the spread of herpes

- Stops the development of colds, colorectal tumors, skin
  cancer, and other types of cancers.

- Effective in killing two strains of melanoma

- Reduces the effects of scarring from radiation treatments

- Decreases the risk of peptic ulcers and may help rid the
  body of the bacteria suspected of causing them

- Benefits the lungs (white wine)
- Lowers levels of type 2 diabetes for postmenopausal women
- Promotes the flow of gastric juices that enhance digestion
- May lower the risk for upper digestive tract cancer
- Reduces cold sores naturally
- Decreases the risk of cataracts
- Fights against periodontal diseases, which attack over 65 percent of senior citizens
- Protects Against Atherosclerosis
- Keeps prostate cells in check
- Reduces stress and depression, kidney acidosis, viruses, and bacteria
- Reduces cholera bacteria
- Reduces e coli bacteria
- Combats typhoid, duodenal ulcers, gall stones, rheumatoid arthritis, osteoporosis, and diabetes mellitus

Is there much left out?

Oh, yes, a recent study posted in 2007 in the *Journal of Agricultural and Food Chemistry* discovered that polyphenols, chemicals present in large amounts in fermented seeds and skins that are cast away after grapes are pressed, interfere with the ability of bacteria to contribute to tooth decay.

Researchers worked with the grape samples of wineries from west-central New York's Finger Lakes, along with the University of Rochester Medical Center and Cornell

University. They exposed *Streptococcus mutans* (which produces a tooth-decaying acid called glucan which causes plaque) that was resistant to the mouth's antibodies to extracts from grapes and grape pomace (wine-making residue) and found that phenolic extracts reduce the essential virulence traits of streptococcus by 70 percent to 85 percent, but don't kill it.

So keep your eyes open in the near future for, who knows, maybe a vino rosso mouth wash.

The study may also hold clues for new ways to reduce life-threatening, systemic infections caused by bacteria.

"Scientists looking for ways to help treat fatty livers have discovered that an ingredient in red wine can help protect from—and possibly even be used to treat—fat buildup in the liver that goes hand-in-hand with chronic alcohol use." 16

And did you know that the majority of cardiovascular physicians treating heart patients allow patients moderate amounts of red wine in their daily diet?

"Moderate drinkers may be less likely to develop blockages in the arteries that supply blood to the legs. In a study of almost 4,000 people over 55, Dutch researchers found that all women and non-smoking men who reported having 1 or 2 drinks a day were less likely than nondrinkers to have peripheral arterial disease (PAD). These results complement previous research that suggests light drinking can reduce cardiovascular disease risk.

"The strongest effect was noted in non-smoking women who were 59% less likely to have PAD than teetotalers.

PAD occurs when arteries in the legs become blocked by a buildup of fatty material, a process known as atherosclerosis. PAD can lead to leg cramps when walking. Atherosclerosis in general can bring on stroke and heart attacks. Alcohol may slow atherosclerosis by inhibiting the oxidation of cholesterol, which prevents it from accumulating inside arteries. Since atherosclerosis can lead to other cardiovascular problems, reducing this process may be the means by which light drinking promotes heart and blood vessel health in general. The benefits of alcohol may stem primarily from red wine. This could explain the stronger effect seen in women, since women tended to choose wine, whereas almost half of men liked beer best." [17]

Are you convinced yet?

Chapter 6

WINE AND BEAUTY

Did it all begin with Cleopatra bathing in wine or mixing it in her skin creams to keep her beauty? Maybe, but we know that using grapes in cosmetology dates as far back as at least the seventeenth century and the court of the French King Louis XIV.

At that time, it was known to French winemakers that aged wine gave a mystical glow when applied to the facial skin. It was the style of that era.

Nowadays, the first In Hollywood to try wine beauty therapy (now labeled vinotherapy throughout international spas) were Julia Roberts and Jennifer Lopez. I guess that started a new trend around the world. It has also led many prestigious cosmetic companies to include the benefits of wine in their products.

By now, you should know the magic bullet in the wine that gives it healing power. Give up?

It's the grape seed.

And do you know what's hidden in this tiny little seed? I gave the answer away in a previous chapter. It's polyphenols, which contain a rich amount of vitamin E that helps the skin to effectively fight off free radicals, which are responsible for wrinkles and skin aging. They also improve circulation by strengthening blood vessels and promoting cell renewal. These radicals are 80 percent responsible for aging.

The antioxidants from grape seeds are fifty times more effective than vitamin E in fighting free radicals and are twenty times more powerful than vitamin C.

These remedies just go on and on.

Leave it to wine to make you beautiful!

Wine soaps, organic shampoos, skin creams, baths, perfumes, fragrances, lotions and potions, antiaging cream, and colognes are used in the vinotherapy process. I must confess, I have never had the pleasure of visiting a spa for vinotherapy.
But I can't wait to try it. And you should too.

Here are a few vinotherapy spas to start with…

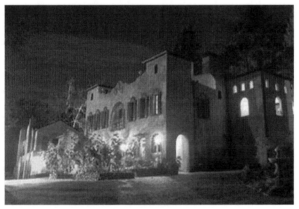

Kenwood Inn and Spa

Sonoma, California
Nation's leading wine spa. A true fantasy for health-conscious wine lovers.

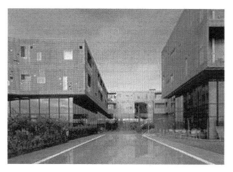

© Loisium Hotel

The Aveda Spa, just a one-hour drive from Vienna, Austria. You can relax in the Barrique Bath and Body Wrap for starters. Next you can try a fine grape facial. Twelve treatment rooms to choose from.

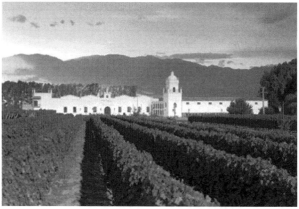

Patios de Cafayate Hotel and Spa

Salta, Argentina
19th-Century Colonial Mansio Spa overlooking trellised vineyards and working wine farm in the Calchaqui' Valley wine region. For more information:
www.starwoodhotels.com

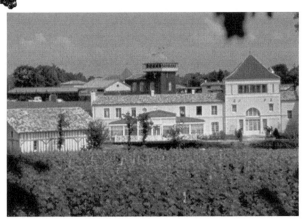

© Les Sources de Caudalie
Bordeaux, France
The world's original vinotherapy spa in the Château Smith Haut-Lafitte vineyards in Bordeaux. For more information: www.sources-caudalie.com.

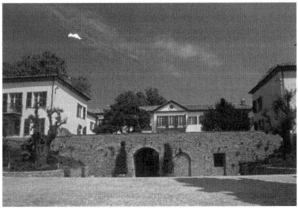

© Relais San Maurizio
San Maurizio, Italy
Found on a hilltop in Italy's Piedmont wine region. Caudalie's second wine therapy spa is part of a seventeenth-century monastery with thirty-one rooms that is a Relais

and Chateau hotel. For more information:
www.relaissanmaurizio.it.

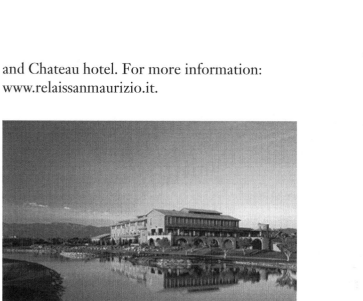

Peralada Resort and Wine Spa

Girona, Spain
This wine spa is a fifty-five-room, Roman-style resort using
grapes, vines, and clays from northern Catalonia's resurgent
Empordà wine region. For more information:
www.golfperalada.com.

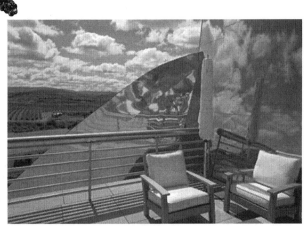

Hotel Marqués de Riscal

Rioja, Spain
Treatments include a hydromassage Red Vine Bath and a classic grapeseed oil Caudalie grand facial that soothes and sculpts the skin. For more information: www.marquesderiscal.com.

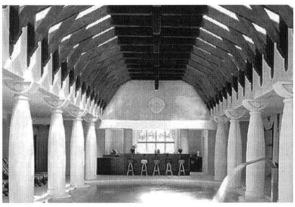

Santé Winelands Hotel and Wellness

Centre, Paarl Valley, South Africa
A ninety-room, Mediterranean-style retreat on a working wine farm outside Cape Town. Offers a signature three-

hour grape cure treatment that involves a shiraz grape seed scrub, a chardonnay cocoon wrap, and a massage, followed by a hydrobath in cabernet. For more information: www.santewellness.com.

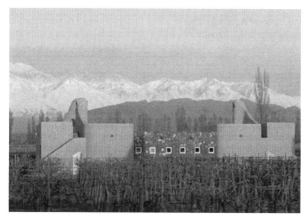

© Cavas Wine Lodge

Mendoza, Argentina
Family-run boutique lodge located in vineyards with views of the Andes in the Mendoza wine country. It offers a vinotherapy pack in a full-service spa.
For more information: www.cavaswinelodge.com.

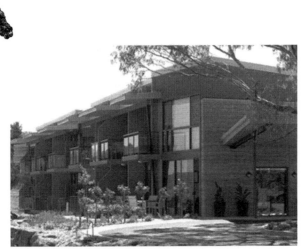

Balgownie Estate Vineyard Resorts and Spa

Yarra Valley, Australia
Indulge yourself with luxurious beauty and spa treatments including massage therapies.
For more information: www.balgownieestate.com.au.

Additional list of Spas around the world:

Silver Star Mountain Resort and Spa
British Columbia, Canada
www.beyondwrapture.com/silverstar

Villagio Inn and Spa, Yountville
Napa Valley, California

Tiger Hill Vineyards Resort and Spa
Maharashtra, India

Dulluva
New York City

Shore Club
South Beach Miami, Florida

Touch Salon and Spa
Houston

Starwood Spa Collection
Spa Agio
Redmond, Washington

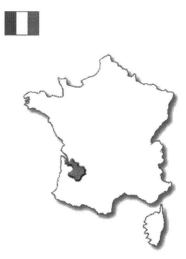

If I were to ask any wine connoisseur what white is the king of all dessert wines, the answer would be Chateau Y'Quem from Bordeaux. And that would be 100 percent correct.

Château d'Yquem
Sauternes
2003

Chateau Y'Quem is known as the finest of all premium dessert wines. If you ever have the pleasure to sip this extraordinary nectar of the gods, you will agree that the wine just melts in your mouth, exemplifying the richness and the concentrate of many fruits lingering on your palate.

It is no wonder that this wine also contains a rich concentration of antioxidants, which have recently been recognized to provide skin benefits too.

No kidding!

Then isn't it fitting that Christian Dior's new eye cream, L' Or de Vie, includes in its ingredients this aristocrat of Bordeaux, Chateau Y'Quem. Some consumers say that it does make a difference and find their skin much smoother and firmer in eight weeks.

It seems the antioxidants from the vine reverse skin damage and aging by stimulating cell and collagen growth.

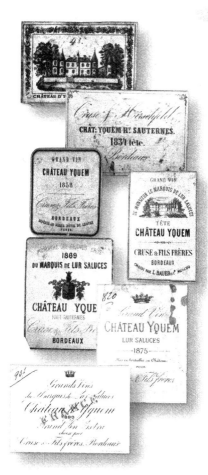

Champagne and Pearl Shampoos
D'Arcy Crushed Pearl Shampoo and Champagne
Conditioner

The conditioner contains champagne and de-oiled French
grape seeds, while the shampoo contains crushed pearl
powder, shea butter, and herbal sunflower.

I can understand the champagne and grape seeds

rejuvenating the hair and the scalp, but where do the crushed pearls fit in?

Granted, everyone's body is different and we all react individually to what we put in it or on it. So before coming to any conclusions, remember, you must try it to find out if it works for you.

Is it possible that baby boomers are living longer by drinking wine which contains resveratrol.

"Harvard researchers are stating this miracle ingredient which helps keep your blood pressure in the normal range, helps with heart health, and better controls the aging process. Resveratrol could be the biggest medical breakthrough in 30 years. In fact, some are calling it the 'Fountain of Youth." [18]

Chapter 7

ORGANIC WINE

As a strong supporter of organic wines and the environment over the years, I tip my hat to Noble Peace Prize winner Al Gore for helping us realize we can all make a difference for a greener Earth. In the wine industry, we have come a long way to the sophisticated palate.

We've had the eco-vine at our fingertips for years, producing the best organic grapes Mother Earth can grow, and only a small percentage of hardworking winemakers believed in growing these grapes and not destroying the soil to produce the true "nectar of the gods."

From a few small wineries producing wines organically to well-known master winemakers bottling some of their best award-winning wines from organic grapes, you can now see the trend spreading. OK, you may pay a slightly higher price for these wines, but you're used to paying a little more for organic produce. Aren't you?

Do you know the old saying that goes something like "I wish I had a nickel every time I was asked that question"? Well, I'm upping the ante to a glass of organic wine every time someone tells me he or she can't drink wine because he or she is allergic to the sulfites.

"They give me a headache" or "I break out in a rash," these people say. These statements go on and on. And everyone blames it on the sulfites.

True, the Food and Drug Administration (FDA) says about 0.4 percent of the population is highly allergic to sulfites. Some people are even sensitive to the natural sulfites found in wine. But migraine headaches are not only from the sulfites; they are also from too many tannins in the wine. White wine contains more sulfites; red wine contains many more tannins.

In fact, I'll bet you that 90 percent of all these claims are self-diagnosed and not the results of medical tests on these individuals.

The U.S. government makes it mandatory that wine producers include a label that reads "Contains Sulfites" on every bottle of wine sold in the United States that has added sulfites (higher than one hundred parts per million). That's the majority of most wines produced, except wines labeled "wine made from organically grown grapes," whose sulfite contents fall under U.S. Department of Agriculture regulations.

So if an individual experiences any type of disorder when drinking wine, it is always blamed on the sulfites.

Hello!

Do you fall into this category?

Have you ever tried a glass of organic wine? It's healthy— try it, you'll like it!

To be called an organic wine, it must be made from organically grown grapes. The soil and plant must be free of herbicides, all synthetic products, chemical fertilizers, and pesticides.

National Organics Program

According to the USDA (United States Department of Agriculture) and the National Organic Program, organic wine is defined as "a wine made from organically grown grapes and without any added sulfites."

This is an ongoing thorn in the side of U.S. wineries that have been calling their wines "organic wines," and now must refer to them as "wines made from organic grapes" or "organically grown grapes," which are allowed to contain a maximum of 100 ppm (parts per million) of added sulfites.

Note: Although it's possible to make a sulfite-free wine with conventional (nonorganic) grapes, it does not qualify as an organic wine.

A certified independent member of the USDA accredits organic wines. He controls each winegrower's abiding by the standards set forth for organic farming. This accreditation can take place once or twice a year.

Organic farming is a traditional belief and method that brings the very best product and taste to the consumer.

Although some producers claim to follow the standards of traditional farming methods, they seem to stray when following the set standards, such as not using synthetic chemicals like fungicides and pesticides or not registering with a legally qualified certification agency.
Caveat emptor: Let the buyer beware!

It is very important for the consumer to be aware that some growers will say their grapes are organic without certification.

As my grandma used to say, "Show me. I want to see it in writing!"

When purchasing wines made from organic grapes, make sure you look for the seal of authenticity from an organic wine certification member in that particular wine region. Label certifications and seals vary internationally. But you can be assured that they follow the same standards and tradition.

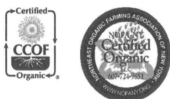

Why is certification extremely important? Because it protects the consumers from fraud!

I've only been in the wine industry for the past forty years, and I can tell you that it was in the late sixties that I stumbled upon organic wines. I was always curious why all vineyards didn't practice this method. I guess, just like anything else, if it's new, people don't understand it. It was

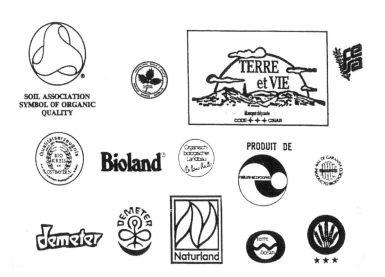

taboo, even if it was healthy for you.

At that time, the entire wine industry was changing from producing bulk wine to varietals. It was unheard of to produce and bottle large quantities of organic wine, especially when the organic vineyards were the size of a postage stamp.

As years went on and organic produce became more and more exposed as a good thing, organic wineries followed the trend. European countries were certifying organic wines within their regions, and more and more wineries followed suit.

I was very surprised to see Champagne, Bordeaux, and other French wine regions with organic certifications, and Italy, Germany, and Spain as well.

In the past two decades, you could probably count on your fingertips the number of reputable organic winegrowers and varietal wines available to the public. I am happy to say that today you can find organic wines made from just about any varietal grape. If you search hard, you may even find the wine region you like producing your favorite wine organically.

Here are images of labels from Organic Wineries & Wine Companies.

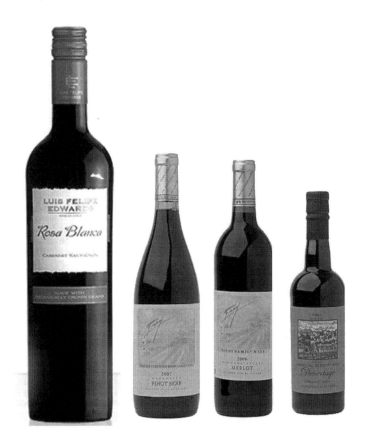

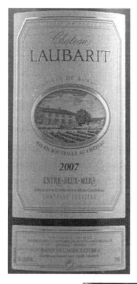

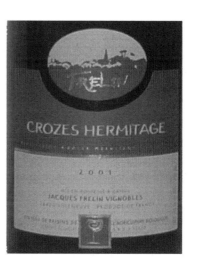

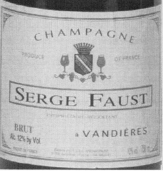

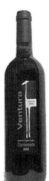

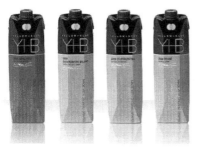

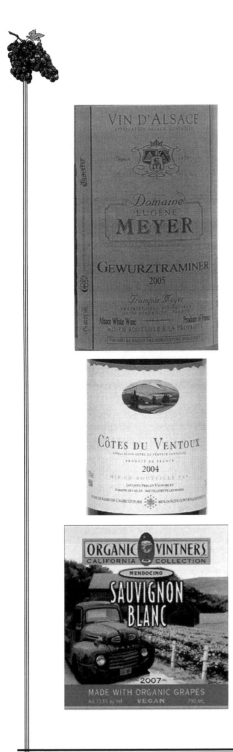

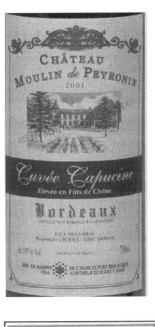

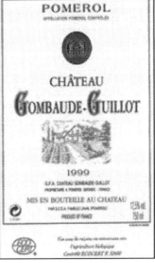

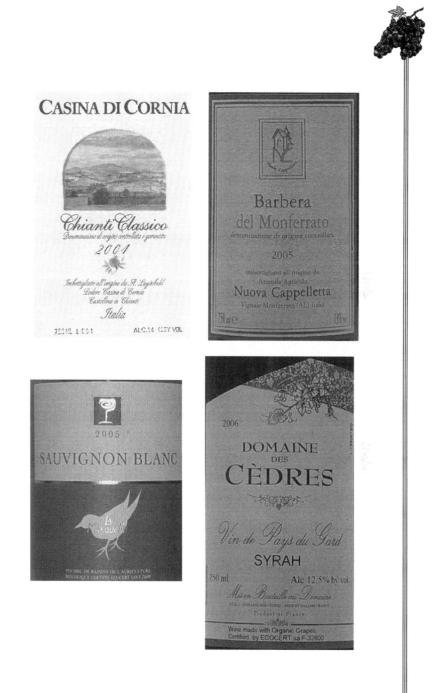

CASINA DI CORNIA

Chianti Classico
Denominazione di origine controllata e garantita

2004

Imbottigliato all'origine da A. Lagerbahl
Podere Casina di Cornia
Castellina in Chianti
Italia

750ML L 001   ALC.14.1 BY VOL

Barbera
del Monferrato
denominazione di origine controllata

2005

imbottigliato all'origine da
Azienda Agricola
Nuova Cappelletta
Vignale Monferrato (AL) Italia

750 cl e   13% vol

2005

SAUVIGNON BLANC

VIN FINE DE RAISINS DE L'AGRICULTURE
BIOLOGIQUE CERTIFIE ECOCERT SAS F-2009

2006

DOMAINE
DES
CÈDRES

Vin de Pays du Gard
SYRAH

750 ml   Alc 12.5% by vol.

Mis en Bouteille au Domaine
EARL DOMAINE DES CEDRES · 30890 SALAZAC FRANCE
Produce of France

Wine made with Organic Grapes
Certified by ECOCERT sa F-32600

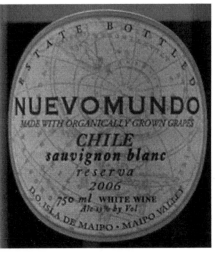

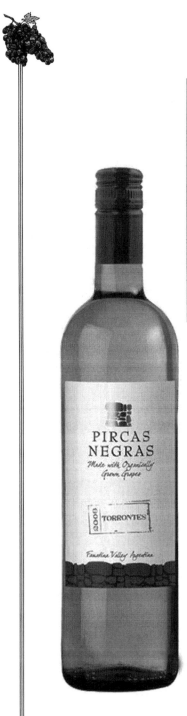

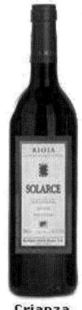

Crianza

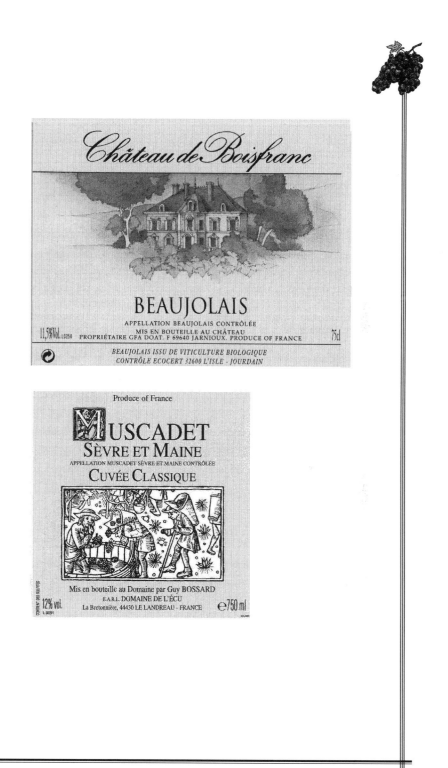

Château de Boisfranc

BEAUJOLAIS

APPELLATION BEAUJOLAIS CONTRÔLÉE
MIS EN BOUTEILLE AU CHÂTEAU
PROPRIÉTAIRE GFA DOAT. F 69640 JARNIOUX. PRODUCE OF FRANCE

11,5% Vol. L0250   75cl

BEAUJOLAIS ISSU DE VITICULTURE BIOLOGIQUE
CONTRÔLE ECOCERT 32600 L'ISLE - JOURDAIN

Produce of France

MUSCADET
SÈVRE ET MAINE
APPELLATION MUSCADET SÈVRE ET MAINE CONTRÔLÉE
CUVÉE CLASSIQUE

Mis en bouteille au Domaine par Guy BOSSARD
E.A.R.L. DOMAINE DE L'ÉCU
La Bretonnière, 44430 LE LANDREAU - FRANCE   ℮ 750 ml

12% vol.
L.9051

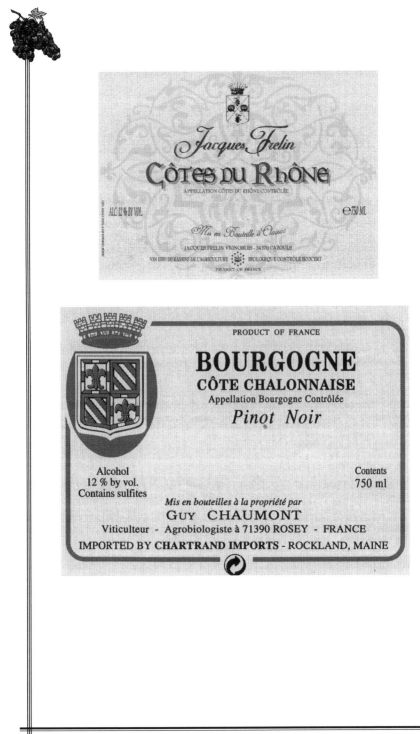

Jacques Frelin

CÔTES DU RHÔNE

APPELLATION CÔTES DU RHÔNE CONTRÔLÉE

ALC. 12 % BY VOL.   ℮ 750 ML

Mis en Bouteille à Claisac

JACQUES FRELIN VIGNOBLES - 34370 CAZOULS

VIN ISSU DE RAISINS DE L'AGRICULTURE BIOLOGIQUE CONTRÔLE ECOCERT
PRODUCT OF FRANCE

PRODUCT OF FRANCE

BOURGOGNE
CÔTE CHALONNAISE
Appellation Bourgogne Contrôlée
Pinot Noir

Alcohol   Contents
12 % by vol.   750 ml
Contains sulfites

Mis en bouteilles à la propriété par
GUY CHAUMONT
Viticulteur - Agrobiologiste à 71390 ROSEY - FRANCE
IMPORTED BY **CHARTRAND IMPORTS** - ROCKLAND, MAINE

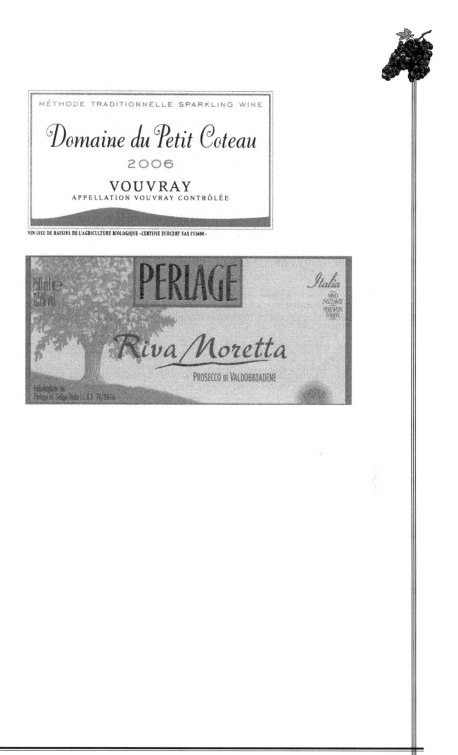

MÉTHODE TRADITIONNELLE SPARKLING WINE

Domaine du Petit Coteau

2006

VOUVRAY
APPELLATION VOUVRAY CONTRÔLÉE

VIN ISSU DE RAISINS DE L'AGRICULTURE BIOLOGIQUE - CERTIFIE ECOCERT SAS F32600 -

PERLAGE

Italia
VINO
FRIZZANTE

PERLWEIN
ITALIEN

750 ml e
11.5% vol

Riva Moretta

PROSECCO DI VALDOBBIADENE

Imbottigliato da
Perlage srl Soligo Italia I.C.R.F. TV/8876

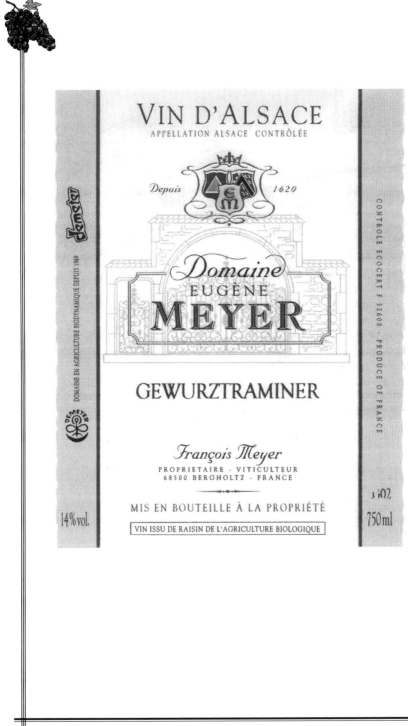

VIN D'ALSACE
APPELLATION ALSACE CONTRÔLÉE

Depuis 1620

Domaine
EUGÈNE
MEYER

GEWURZTRAMINER

François Meyer
PROPRIETAIRE - VITICULTEUR
68500 BERGHOLTZ · FRANCE

MIS EN BOUTEILLE À LA PROPRIÉTÉ

VIN ISSU DE RAISIN DE L'AGRICULTURE BIOLOGIQUE

14 % vol.

750 ml

DOMAINE EN AGRICULTURE BIODYNAMIQUE DEPUIS 1969

CONTROLE ECOCERT F 32600 · PRODUCE OF FRANCE

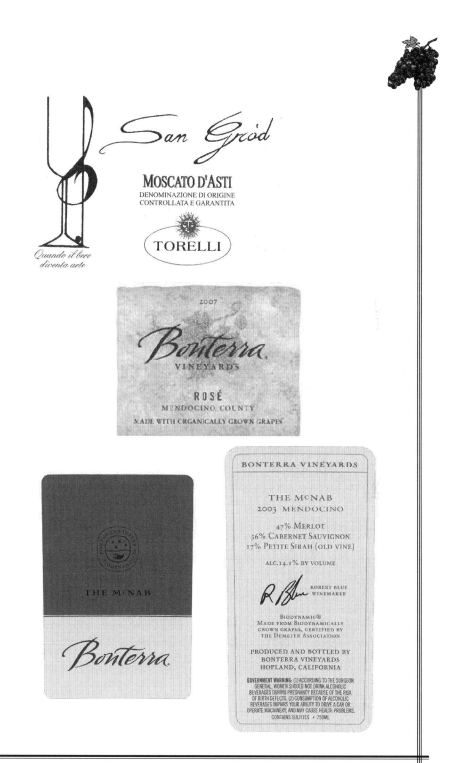

San Gród

MOSCATO D'ASTI
DENOMINAZIONE DI ORIGINE
CONTROLLATA E GARANTITA

TORELLI

*Quando il bere
diventa arte*

2007

Bonterra
VINEYARDS

ROSÉ
MENDOCINO COUNTY
MADE WITH ORGANICALLY GROWN GRAPES

THE McNAB

Bonterra.

BONTERRA VINEYARDS

THE McNAB
2003 MENDOCINO

47% MERLOT
36% CABERNET SAUVIGNON
17% PETITE SIRAH (OLD VINE)

ALC.14.1% BY VOLUME

ROBERT BLUE
WINEMAKER

BIODYNAMIC®
MADE FROM BIODYNAMICALLY
GROWN GRAPES, CERTIFIED BY
THE DEMETER ASSOCIATION

PRODUCED AND BOTTLED BY
BONTERRA VINEYARDS
HOPLAND, CALIFORNIA

GOVERNMENT WARNING: (1) ACCORDING TO THE SURGEON
GENERAL, WOMEN SHOULD NOT DRINK ALCOHOLIC
BEVERAGES DURING PREGNANCY BECAUSE OF THE RISK
OF BIRTH DEFECTS. (2) CONSUMPTION OF ALCOHOLIC
BEVERAGES IMPAIRS YOUR ABILITY TO DRIVE A CAR OR
OPERATE MACHINERY, AND MAY CAUSE HEALTH PROBLEMS.
CONTAINS SULFITES • 750ML.

Here is a list of organic wineries and wine companies where you can begin your search.

ARIZONA

Kokopelliwinery

CALIFORNIA

A

Andersen Vineyards (Santa Cruz)

B

Barra Of Mendocino (Redwood Valley)
Benziger Family Winery (Glen Ellen)
Beringer Vineyards (St. Helena)
Bonterra Vineyards (Ukiah)
Buena Vista Carneros (Sonoma)

C

Casa Barranca Winery (Ojai)
Ceago Winegarden (Nice)
Charles Krug (St.Helena)
Clos Pepe Vineyards (Lompoc)
Coates Vineyards (Orleans)
Coturri Winery (Glen Ellen)

D

Davis Bynum Winery (Healdsburg)
De Tierra Vineyards (Salinas)
Del Bondio Wine Company (Napa)

E

Ehlers Estate (St. Helena)

Everett Ridge Vineyards & Winery (Healdsburg)

F

Fasi Estate Vineyard (Madera)
Fetzer Vineyards (Hopland)
Fitzpatrick Winery & Lodge (Fair Play)
Five Rivers Winery (Paso Robles)
Four Gates Winery (Kosher/Santa Cruz)
Frey Vineyards (Redwood Valley)

G

Gorasole Vineyards

H

Hallcrest Vineyards (Felton)
Heller Estate (Carmel Valley)
Herzog Wine Cellars (Kosher/Oxnard)
Honeyrun Winery (Chico)

J

Jorian Hill Vineyards (Solvang)
Jeriko Estate

K

Kaz Vineyard & Winery (Kenwood)

L

La Rocca Vineyards (Forest Ranch)
Lavender Ridge Vineyard (Murphys)
La Vie Vineyards (Lompoc)
Le Vin Vineyards & Winery (Yorkville)
Long Meadow Ranch (St. Helena)

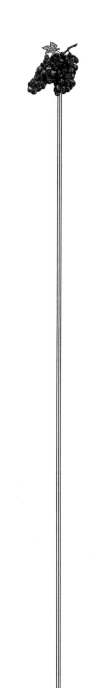

M

Madonna Estate (Napa)
Marimar Estate (Sebastopol)
Mcevoy Ranch (Petaluma)
Medlock Ames (Healdsburg)
Montemaggiore (Healdsburg)
Muir- Hanna Vineyards (Napa)
Murphy Creek Vineyards (Clements)
Murray's Cyder (Forestville)

N

Napa Wine Company
Nevada County Wine Guild (Nevada City)

O

Old World Winery (Windsor)
Organic Vintages (Ukiah)
Organic Wine Company (San Francisco)
Oster Wine Cellars (Redwood Valley)

P

Pavi Wines (Oakville)
Presidio Vineyard & Winery (Lompoc)
Preston Vineyards (Healdsburg)

Q

Quivira Vineyards (Healdsburg)

R

Retzlaff Winery (Livermore)
Richard Grant Wine (Napa)
Robert Mondavi Winery (Oakville)
Robert Sinskey Vineyards (Napa)

S

Silver Mountain Vineyards (Santa Cruz)
Smith Vineyard (Grass Valley)
Spottswoode Vineyards (Livermore)
Sunce' Winery (Santa Rosa)
Sunstone Vineyards & Winery (Santa Ynez)

T

Tablas Creek Vineyard (Paso Robles)
Teachworth Cabs (Calistoga)
Topolos At Russian River (Forestville)

V

Vine Cliff Winery (Napa)
Volker Eisele Family Estate (St. Helena)

W

Wente Vineyards (Livermore)
White Rock Vineyards (Napa)
Wild Hog Vineyard (Graton)
Winnett Vineyards (Willow Creek)

Y

Yorkville Cellars (Yorkville)

MAINE

Chartrand Importers (Rockland)

NEW YORK

Four Chimneys (Himrod)

OREGON

Copper Mountain
Maysara
Sokol Blosser

WASHINGTON

Badger Mountain Wine
K Vintners

AUSTRIA

Hafner Winery

FRANCE

La Marouette
Faust, Champagne

SOUTH AFRICA

Stellar Winery

SPAIN

Nina Bonita Organic Sangria

Organic Wines from around the world:

Guy Chaumont Bourgogne Pinot Noir
Richmond Plains Nelson Pinot Noir
Riva Moretta Prosecco Frizzante
Casina di Cornia Chianti Classico
Mario Torelli Moscato d' Asti "San Grod"
Guy Bossard Muscadet
Chateau de Boisfranc Beaujolais
Jacques Frelin Cote du Rhone
Domaine Du Petit Coteau Sparkling Vouvray
Coturri Pinot Noir Lost Creek Vineyards

NSA Port Badger Mountain
Eugene Meyer Alsace Gewurztraminer

Now let's get back to sulfites in the wine!

If you are under the assumption that organic wines contain no sulfites, I have news for you: all wines contain natural sulfites!

Yes, even in organic wines, there is no such thing as a sulfite-free wine. Sulfites are a natural by-product in the fermentation process. During fermentation, the grape skins have a fermenting yeast that naturally generates sulfites. This amount ranges from about 6 to 40.

Although most organic wines contain less than 40 ppm of sulfites, in the United States, nonorganic wines can contain up to 350 ppm of sulfites. The USDA limits organic winemaking standards of added sulfites to 100 ppm in all finished products.

Note: Organic wines have fewer sulfites than conventional wine. Therefore, when opened, they will not last long, should you decide to leave wine in the bottle for another day. I also suggest that you check the vintage on the bottle before purchase. Organic wines should be consumed young, within a year. These wines are not recommended for storing in a wine cellar.

Wine Tip

When I have wine left over in a bottle, I like to preserve it by using a Vacu Vin style pump. It's very easy to use and it does the trick. It costs less than $14 and it usually comes with two rubber corks, each with a slit through the middle from top to bottom. After you fit the rubber cork in the bottle, you place the pump over the cork and pump it a few times. This will remove the air in the bottle through the slit sealing the cork. When you decide to drink the contents, just squeeze the cork a little and remove. It's as easy as that. And it will preserve the wine for a least a week. Make sure you store the wine in a cool area.

CHAPTER 8

VEGAN WINES

Here's a little trick I play…I like to ask vegetarians (over twenty-one) if they drink wine. Nine times out of ten, people answer yes! Then I ask, what kind of wine do you drink? Answer: all kinds.

That's when I put them into shock…

I begin by saying, "Did you know that most of the wine you are drinking includes agents of animal origin?"

That's when they lose it!

All the years of proclaiming they are vegetarians are washed down the drain. I usually let them sweat a few seconds before telling them that there are all types of vegan wines available. Most vegetarians have never heard of vegan wines, and they ask where they can buy them.

You can purchase them in most fine wine shops. Plain and simple, if your favorite wine shop has a good selection of wine, the proprietor should be aware of specialty wines like organic, vegan, and biodynamic wines. If you can't find these wines in your favorite shop, they can be ordered and delivered through their distributor within forty-eight hours.

In simple terms, to qualify as a vegan wine, no animal-derived products can be used in the production of the wine. They are instead clarified with kaolin or bentonite clay minerals. This decision of what to use in the production is entirely up to the winemaker. Some prefer to filter manually without using any additives.

One of the techniques used by winemakers producing organic or nonorganic wine is using animal products in "fining" or clearing the wine. In some European countries years ago, these products consisted of fish oil, egg whites, and oxen's or bull's blood, which were inexpensive and convenient. Now don't get excited; this practice is now illegal in most countries since the outbreak of BSE (bovine spongiform encephalopathy—mad cow disease).

The filtering process prevents the wine from becoming cloudy. Fining also removes the bad tastes and flavors in the early stage of production.
Some organic wine producers use gelatin. The most powerful of the organic fining, gelatin will also remove excess tannins (polyphenolics) and coloring particles (melanoidins) from wine.

Note: If you find a vintage vegan wine that you enjoy, it is not set in stone that the next vintage of the same wine will be a vegan wine. The decision in "fining" with or without animal by-products is at the discretion of the winemaker. It is always a good idea to check with the winery before purchasing.

Here are just a few vegan wines to start with:

ARGENTINA

Pircas Negras

AUSTRALIA

Cranswick, Shiraz / Cabernet
Jarrah Ridge, Chardonnay
Palandri, Australian Red

CALIFORNIA

Jack Rabbit, Pinot Grigio
Organic Vineyards, Sauvignon Blanc
Turn Stone, California Red

CHILE

Nuevo Mundo, Sauvignon Blanc & Cabernet Sauvignon

ENGLAND (Holy Island)

Real Fruit Wine
Lanchester, Blackberry & Apple
Lanchester, Strawberry
Lanchester Ginger & Fruit

FRANCE

Serge Faust, Champagne
Blanquette De Limoux, Methode Traditionelle Sparkling
Guy Chaumont, Borgogne Cote Chalonnaise
Domaine des Cedres, Cote du Rhone
Chateau Moulin de Peyronin, Bordeaux
Chateau Laubarit, Entre Deux Mers

Lamaraquette, Cabernet Sauvignon
Meyer, Gewurtstraminer, Alsace
Andre Bourguet, Cartegne Vin de Liqueur (Dessert)

GERMANY

Villa Wolf Pinot Gris

ITALY

Botter Valpolicella
Colli Vicentini Pinot Grigio, Veneta
Del Monferrato Barbera (Piemonte)

NEW ZEALAND

Southern Lights Sauvignon Blanc, Marlborough
Kono Sauvignon Blanc
Wright wines

PORTUGAL

CJ Casal Black Label Porto
Cordovero Porto

SOUTH AFRICA

Cape Bay Chenin Blanc, Pinotage,
Neil Joubert Merlot

SPAIN

Solarce Blanco Tinto, Rosado Ecologico–Crianza-Rioja
Vina Ardenza Tinto Reserva
La Vicalanda Gran Reserva
Sherry:
Jose de Sota Pale Cream, Fino, Amontillado
Vegan Tio Pepe, Palomino Fino (Pale)

UNITED KINGDOM

Sedlescombe English Organic Wines

UNITED STATES

Fitzpatrick Organic Winery,
Frey Vineyards of California Organic Wine Works of
California

Did you know…

All kosher wine is 100 percent vegan. Due to strict Jewish
laws, all wine must be made without any animal by-products
whatsoever—no meat, fish, dairy, or eggs—so kosher wine is
always a great choice for vegans!

Biodynamic Wine Labels

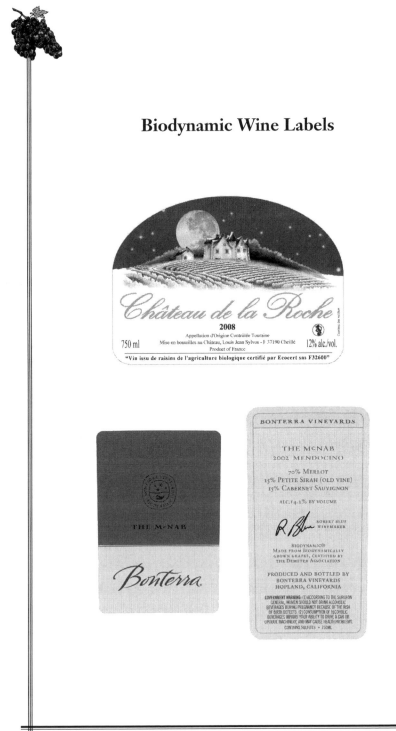

Chapter 9

BIODYNAMIC WINES

It is written that wine has been around for more than four thousand years. I would love to have tasted a wine from biblical times.

I can only dream and imagine tasting a wine from grapes grown on a vine in virgin, balanced soil absorbing the minerals and nutrients that reflect in the finished product. Very similar is the biodynamic agriculture method of making a healthy wine. All biodynamic wine is 100 percent organic.

Biodynamics takes organic grape growing and winemaking a few steps further. The biodynamic method is a little bit spiritual in nature, a practical philosophy (anthroposophy) understanding the ecological, energetic, and mystical balancing in the grape-growing nature of the terroir.

Grape growers who have tried the biodynamic method have found a quick improvement in their vineyards— improvement in the soil fertility, crop nutrition, disease management, and insect and weed control. They have also found the wines to be stronger and longer lasting than the organic wines.

These wines are made with no added sulfites. Innovative winemaking techniques compensate for the lack of this pungent preservative (which can, as we've mentioned, induce headaches, sniffles, and other allergic reactions in people).

The wine is therefore free to reveal its delicate and true flavors. Emphasis is on producing wine of the highest quality while caring for planet and palate alike. If you have never had the opportunity to taste a biodynamic wine, I strongly recommend that you do. It will be one of your greatest wine experiences.

After all, the most expensive wine in the world, Romanée-Conti, (Burgundy District of France) is biodynamic!

Bonterra Vineyards of Mendocino
Fitzpatrick Organic Winery
Frey Vineyards of California
Organic Wineworks of California.
Sedlescombe English organic wines
Reyneke, South Africa
Wright Wines in New Zealand

Chapter 10

ORGANIC SAKÉ

Is saké brewed, similar to beer making, or is it fermented and made like wine? I guess you can say a little bit of both.

If you didn't already know it, saké is made from rice. I'm not talking about Uncle Ben's minute rice. It takes a lot more time, hard work, and dedication to make an excellent-tasting organic saké.

Whether drinking saké from Japan or any other country, with the word "organic" on the label, you know the producer takes the product one step further to assure customers they are getting a product made with the very best care.

Saké has many health benefits, and organic saké just adds more proof to benefit the human body.

To begin with, we know that osteoporosis is an incurable disease that makes bones brittle, and there is no specific medical treatment. Researchers have found that women can prevent osteoporosis by the use of certain female hormones. Studies have shown that allergy inhibitors in saké koji can help fight osteoporosis inhibitors for those who drink three to six small glasses a week in moderation.

Saké drinking in moderation? Seems like we are finding similar preventatives as we found in my early chapters for drinking red and white wine.

Did you know that saké contains many elements, including amino acids, which are good for stimulating brain functioning and help to prevent cancer at the same time?

As you read on, it is important to know that it is the by-product after the pressing of the last pure drop (the lees) that scientists say is responsible for activating the natural killer cell (kind of lymphocyte) known to kill only cancer cells.

More proven data from Japanese scientists claim that saké is shown to be very effective in increasing good cholesterol and producing better blood flow. This takes us a few steps further: saké is also very effective in dissolving thrombi (fatty tissues) in arteries.

Let's not forget my searching for the fountain of youth. Can saké be our guide to preventing aging and Alzheimer's disease (AD)? Researchers have stated that saké is very effective in preventing forgetfulness as well. Moderate saké drinkers have better brain functioning than people who don't drink at all.

As I always said, I don't condone drinking alcoholic beverages, but if you're worried about cirrhosis of the liver, you may take this into account: doctors have stated the reason the liver does not function well in cirrhosis patients is the difficulty in processing protein. Drinking saké, which contains amino acids, in moderation can help to ensure good health.

If you would like to try an organic Nama Saké, I recommend Sho Chiku Bai (NAMA SAKÉ) made with organic rice. Produced and bottled by Takara Saké USA, Inc. This organic saké is the first saké in the United States (California) produced from organic rice. This draft-type

Nama Saké is a delicious, full-bodied saké with a hint of fruity aromas. Its mild, smooth, and fresh taste pairs well with a wide range of foods, from sushi to teriyaki dishes. Look for a green frosted bottle with the certified organic OCIA seal on the bottle.

If you haven't tried the new styles of saké, I suggest you do. Whether tasting it hot or cold, I'm sure you will find a type that fits your needs. If you get the chance, don't leave out sparkling saké. It's worth the experience.

The following is the stages of producing Saké.

Saké Rice - Sakamai

The rice is planted in May and June and harvested in August and September. Similar to wine vintages there are good years and bad years for Saké rice and the weather plays a very important part . Although Japan gets Typhoons and excessive rain which could be the biggest obstacle, master saké makers can adjust to these conditions and still produce saké of excellent quality.

Rice Polishing – Seimai

The first stage in making Saké, brewers mill the rice to its heart. This process is called seimi or rice-polishing (Seimaibuai) . Let's compare it to polishing a diamond. There are different layers or levels of Saké. When you mill the rice you remove the fats, proteins and amino acids from the outer level of the rice grain. Leaving the starch filled center untouched which makes the saké more refined and elegant as a diamond.

Rinsing - Senmai

When the rice is milled the first layer of rice powder is used for feeding animals. In the beginning you will find the rice brown in color and also the powder. The powder produced in the next stage of milling is use to make food products, such as rice crackers (sembe).

After this stage of milling the Saké makers rinse the rice that is left on the grain. At the same time the rice is also soaked to remove the powder. Now the rice is ready for the next stage, steaming. This is a very crucial time because depending on the type of rice and its milling level, rinsing and soaking are done with the precision of, and I'm not kidding, a stop watch.

Steaming - Jomai

Did you know that Saké rice is not boiled like table rice. Saké makers steam in a koshiki and if the rice is not carefully steamed enough it could turn out too hard for the next stage to be correct. Here again, just like a celler masters skill in making wine, the saké maker must be very careful not to over steam the rice or it will become mushy, which makes it very difficult for certain necessary enzymes to fully produce. When steaming is complete the rice is then allowed to cool. Here twenty to thirty percent of steam rice is used for koji, the remainder is mixed in with the koji rice at the beginning of brewing or fermentation.

Koji Making

Very similar to the room used for fermenting wine, the room in which koji is made is called the muro, this is the heart of the brewery. I know your saying to yourself. What is Koji? It's a mold that converts the complex sugars in rice into simple sugars. In making koji rice the brewers sprinkle koji powder on a portion of the steamed rice. Then the process begins. During the next 40-plus hours, they knead, wrap, unwrap, spread out and cool this rice. By the end of this process, the rice is 100 percent simple sugar and has a white, frost like coating.

Some may say that the aroma is very similar to roasted chestnuts. In the beginning of this chapter I asked the question is Saké brewed like beer or fermented like wine. Have you decided yet? Here is some more information to help you decide.

"Saké Mother" (Shubo) or "Foundation" (Moto)

These are the names of the yeast starters which reflect the importance of this step. The yeast starter is a highly concentrated "mini batch" of Saké made up of koji rice, water, yeast and steamed rice. There are three ways to make yeast starter, kimoto (the original way), yamahai (the second way) and sokujo (the modern,fast way).

There are also 50 different kinds of saké yeast, with 15 major types. Some were developed in certain regions, others by particular breweries; some yield light and refined saké, others bolder and more intense flavors.

Three-step brewing - San-dan shikomi

When they make this concentrate, the brewers start the fermentation process by adding these ingredients three times, multiplying the amounts by two each time. This process is called shikomi, the koji rice goes to work on the remaining steamed rice, converting its starches into simple

sugars in a process called "multiple parallel fermentation."
Next the brew is fermented which takes about seventeen to
twenty five days.

Fermentation - Moromi

Before fermentation takes place, all processes of milling,
rinsing, soaking, steaming, making koji, making the moto
and brewing it in three stages, the brew begins the
fermentation. Some may say this process is less laborious,
but the brewers must precisely and repeatedly control this
stage. Fermentation usually takes between 17 to 24 days of
constant overseeing and adjusting.

Pressing – Joso

When fermentation is complete, Saké makers (kurabito)
press the moromi in a large machine that looks like an
accordion called a yabuta. A more specialized process by the
kurabito is to fill cotton bags with the finished brew, which
is then place in a boat shaped object called a fune'. This
allows the fresh brewed Saké to slowly seep out of the bags
at the bottom of the fune'. When the Saké has finished
draining the Saké makers use a flat lid and gently press
down the extra remaining Saké.

The most refined process is called shizuki meaning drops.
This is when brewers hang the cotton bags on bamboo
poles to let the Saké drip into smaller tanks. Shizuku Saké
taste very fresh, light with an elegant taste.

Filtration and Bottling - Roka

Similar to wine making, after pressing, Saké is filtered,
pasteurized twice and stored in bottles, or tanks to be
bottled at a later date. Saké is brewed from the beginning of

October until the end of March which is usually released after six months storing. So, to truly answer my question, "Is saké brewed like beer or fermented like wine? Most of the experts seem to lean towards brewed like beer.

Now that you have an idea of how saké is made, you need to understand that the U.S. has different standards than Japan and they will not alloy Imported Organic Saké to bear the name ORGANIC on the label.

Organic rice is certified by the Japanese Agricultural Standards (JAS) board, under the auspices of the Ministry of Agriculture, Forestry and Fisheries. They must prove that this rice has been grown in a rice paddy where no agricultural chemicals have been used for at least three years and must be certified by a third party.

Presently, organic nihonshu is defined by the Ministry of Taxation as saké in which 95% or more of the rice used in brewing qualifies as JAS-certified organically grown rice.

In Japan there are only a few saké made with organic rice, as of 2009 you will only find one certified organic saké. This would be a junmai ginjo brewed by Saiya Shuzoten of Akita Prefecture. Look for Yuki no Bosha and Yuri Masamune brands. This brewery is the very first saké brewery in Japan to be certified as an organic food and things processing factory. This Yuki no Bosha organic junmai ginjo has been officially certified by the ASAC (Association for Sustainable Agricultural Certification).

One, true organic certification is very stringent and specific. The rice may have been grown with something the brewer or farmer doesn't consider a chemical, which would not be an approved standard method or substance. Remember that the Japanese landscape and water irrigation practices may make it very difficult for a rice paddy to be certified due to a flow down from a higher paddy with chemical practicing from one particular rice field. The rice field itself might not be officially certified as organic, If a producer cannot absolutely guarantee that that water has not been contaminated by chemicals somewhere down the line, it cannot be certified as organic.

This is one more reason saké is sometimes labeled as "munouyaku" and not "organic." So the next time you look for a good Imported Organic Saké look for the above mentioned companies with "high ecological standards" Made the traditional way using the yamahai and kimoto methods.

That brewery, as mentioned above, is called Saiya Shuzoten, and is known for two well-established brands Yuri Masamune, and Yuki no Bosha. Their saké is elegant, with an amazing consistency of fragrance. Their futsuu-shu (table saké) right up to their ginjo all share a similar fragrance and a touch of elegance.

You will find Yuki no Bosha (Akita Prefecture) Junmai Ginjo Organic Saké well balanced, full bodied which reflects the intensity to the flavor. The skill of the kurabito brings out such elegant flavors that there is never an off-flavor of the product. Although the brewer believes this lack of off-flavors is a direct positive result of the organic methods. Domestic

Organic Saké

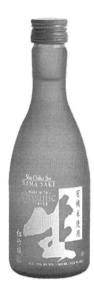

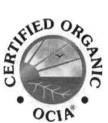

Types of Saké

Saké can be divided into the following groups according to the type of brewing process.

Junmai

The name means "pure rice". Junmai is saké composed of only rice, water, koji and saké yeast. No other ingredients or additives, such as alcohol or sugar, are added. The rice that has been polished to 70% or less of its original size is used to brew. The saké character tends to have a full-bodied and slightly acidic.

Honjozo

In this saké, not more than 120 liters or raw alcohol per each metric ton of white rice and no glucose have been added during brewing process. Added alcohol cannot exceed 25% of the total alcohol in the finished product. In the U.S. it is not legal to make Honjozo or to add alcohol to saké. Imported Honjozo is categorized into distilled spirits. The saké character tends to lighter than Junmai.

Ginjo

Ginjo is a special type of Junmai or Honjozo, and considered the highest achievement of the brewer's art. All the rice employed in brewing Ginjo must be polished to at least 60% of its original size. Dai-Ginjo is brewed with the rice polished to at least 50%. In many Ginjo brewers use special yeasts in making Moto, and ferment the final mash very slowly at low temperature. This extra effort produce a saké that is lighter, clean taste and tangy flavor and an aroma.

Nama

Nama means "Draft saké". In this saké, fresh saké is microfiltered instead of other saké is pasteurized twice, once before aging and once in the process of bottling. Nama is fruity and fresh taste with pleasant aroma.

Nigori

Nigori -"Cloudy"- saké is unfilterd or roughly filterd so that some Moromi in the fermenting tank make it into the bottle. This saké is a milky white appearance. Nigori is bold and sweet taste.

Genshu

Genshu is undiluted saké. After filtration, saké has an alcohol content of around 19%. Most of saké on the market have been diluted with water until their alcohol contents falls to between 12 and 16%. Genshu is full-bodied and rich taste.

If you haven't tried the new styles of saké, I suggest you do. Whether tasting it hot or cold I'm sure you will find a type that fits your needs. If you get the chance, don't leave out sparkling Saké it's worth the expeience.

CHAPTER 11

NON ALCOHOL WINES

Just like it says, non-alcoholic wine. You've heard of it, you've seen it in supermarkets, but I bet you've never tried it.

Is it really nonalcoholic?

Technically, yes, but it is physically impossible to remove 100 percent of the alcohol from any fermented juice.

The legal definition of a nonalcoholic wine requires it to contain less than ½ of 1 percent alcohol.

Some nonalcoholic wine tastes great and is made from popular grape varietals such as chardonnay, Riesling, cabernet sauvignon, merlot, and zinfandel. You can also find nonalcoholic sparkling wines, which reminds me of a sparkling punch recipe my family has been using for years.

Nonalcoholic Sparkling Wine

1 punch bowl
3 bottles nonalcoholic sparkling wine
1 2-liter bottle of ginger ale
10 small balloons, assorted colors

Yes, I said balloons!

Rinse the balloons and fill them with water the night before the party. Do not blow them up. Fill them so they are just about the size of a golf ball and tie them tight. Then freeze them overnight.

The next day, add them to the punch. This will make the bowl colorful and keep the punch cold without diluting the punch.

If you don't want to use balloons to chill the punch, you can fill ice trays with non-alcoholic chardonnay wine, and when they freeze just add them to the punch. This will give your punch added wine flavor.

Another idea is to freeze fruit, such as grapes, strawberries, melon balls, etc. Using frozen fruit can sweeten the taste of the punch, so be careful of the fruit you add.

Nonalcoholic wines are great to cook with because they are less expensive than table wines containing alcohol.

The general rule when cooking is "the better the wine you cook with, the better the food will taste." When you cook with wines that contain alcohol, the alcohol burns off within the first minute, leaving the flavor of the wine. Don't be afraid to taste the wine before you cook with it.

Remember this: good wine tastes good, and bad wine tastes bad. Plain and simple, don't make the mistake of cooking with the wine before you taste it.

If you are looking to purchase a nonalcoholic wine that tastes good, you should look for a wine where the winemaker uses a cold process to remove the alcohol.

Let me explain.

There are two processes used to remove the alcohol from a

beverage. One process is heat or evaporation to remove the alcohol. This process damages the natural flavors of the grape. The second would be a cold process of less than fifty degrees Fahrenheit, which retains all the natural flavors of the grape.

You can find this information by visiting these nonalcoholic wines' Web sites.

CALIFORNIA

arielvineyards.com
sutterhomefre.com

OREGON

drapervalleyvineyard.com
youngberghill.com

PENNSYLVANIA

sandcastlewinery.com

GERMANY

carljungwines.com

Warning:

Many people think that because these wines are labeled nonalcoholic, they can be offered to alcoholics and people who are diagnosed with diabetes or kidney and liver ailments. I say this: for a recovering alcoholic, this is a very personal and sensitive issue, and he or she should not be tempted.

If you are not sure about your medical ailments and nonalcoholic wine, I suggest you first check with your personal physician.

Alcohol or no alcohol in the wine.

That is the question!

Here is one answer:

"There's been a lot of talk lately about avoiding alcohol—the bête noire of many while still preserving the health benefits of wine, a sort of having your antioxidant and not drinking it, too. Grape juice, dealcoholized wine, and resveratrol capsules are being promoted as more temperate, more healthful alternatives to wine. Let's critically examine what alcohol brings, particularly to wine, most particularly to the health of the wine drinker. It should be remembered that drinking wine or any alcoholic drink should be for pleasure and relaxation rather than for any given health benefits, however.

"Alcohol, that is, ethyl alcohol (ethanol), contributes body and flavor to wine and other naturally fermented beverages, helping to preserve and enliven them, and, through its volatility, enables the all-important bouquet to bloom. Medical evidence over the last thirty years shows repeatedly that alcohol itself accounts for at least 50 percent to 60 percent of the many and now-familiar health benefits of moderate wine consumption. Polyphenolic antioxidants take care of most of the remainder. Some of the salubrious effects involve a joint venture between alcohol and polyphenols." [19]

It may not please wine connoisseurs, but red wine without the alcohol is also good for the heart, researchers report. Dr. Jennifer R. C. Bell and colleagues at the University of California, Davis, report the results of their study, in which they took a 1996 cabernet sauvignon and removed the alcohol. They then asked five men and four women—all healthy— to drink about a half cup of the wine, with water added on one day and water and ethanol added on the other. The investigators measured levels of the flavonoid "(+)-catechin" the wine component credited with heart benefits— after consumption.

The researchers collected blood at baseline and then thirty minutes, one hour, two, three, four, and eight hours after consumption. They found that the half-life of (+)-catechin was significantly shorter (3.17 hours) when subjects drank alcoholic red wine than when they drank the dealcoholized version (4.08 hours). Bell and colleagues report that increases in total (+)-catechin in plasma were similar after ingestion of alcoholic and nonalcoholic red wine and that gender had no effect.

But moderate amounts of alcohol also contribute to heart health. Previous research shows that alcohol by itself increases concentration of HDL—"the good cholesterol"— in the blood, the researchers note. "The results (of this study)…suggest that red wine provides two independent factors capable of contributing to vascular health when consumed in moderation," the investigators write, namely the HDL-boosting effects of alcohol and the increase of flavonoids in the blood.

CHAPTER 12

LOW CALORIE WINE

Low-calorie wines have been made to appeal to women, who are credited with about 80 percent of all the wine sales in the United States. This wine category is not entirely new to the wine drinkers who would like to watch their calorie intake a little more closely. Quite a few brands have come and gone. I will tell you this for sure. We're in a health-conscious era, and it seems that once again wine companies are trying to corner the market with their new low-calorie wine creations.

And why not?

Beringer Vineyards of California has produced White Lie Early Season Chardonnay, hoping to appeal to women. Let's not leave out the opposite sex. I decided to take a survey on my own, and you would be surprised how many men watching their calories would try a low-calorie vino.

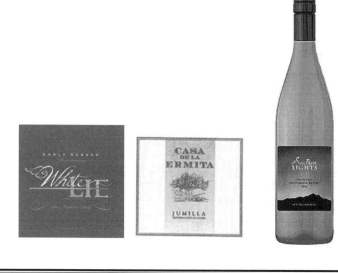

Low-Calorie Wine from Spain

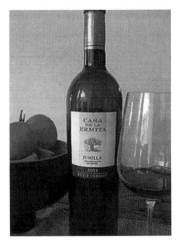

As a result of the drought in Spain, leave it to the Spaniards to produce a new low-calorie red wine. The vineyard in Jumilla, Murcia, with the help of researchers from the Murcia and Cartagena University and the Technological Development Center, which is part of the Ministry for Industry, have come up with the name "vino light." This red 2006 crianza is a blend of three varietal grapes (monastrell, tempranillo, and verdot). The winemakers' technique is to deprive the vine of water for several hours a day while the grapes begin to age, which results in a lower alcohol content (about 6.5 percent), half of the normal amount in still wine. They have invested well over two million dollars in this project, and the wine can now be purchased from your favorite wine shop.

Another low-calorie wine from Spain is Valduero "Sobresaliente" Albillo Vino de Mesa. Bodegas Valduero, located in Gumiel de Mercado, was established in 1984 as the sixth registered bodega of the now 109 in Ribera del

Duero DO. The Garcia family (who own and operate the winery) were among the first to recognize the incredible potential that the Ribera del Duero soils held and started acquiring vineyards and planting vines before the region became internationally recognized. Having two hundred hectares of vineyards allows them to control the quality of the base material and ensure that superior fruit is used for their superior wines. Also, Valduero wines represent an extraordinary value because they own their vineyards and do not have to source their fruit on the ever-rising open market. This low-in-alcohol, new, slimline wine, Sobresaliente, is a Spanish white that boasts just fifty calories—well below the average of eighty calories a glass. Ideal

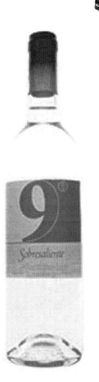

for dieters, one glass has the same number of calories as an apple. You will find this Spanish sleeper, as we call it, very fresh and easy to drink. This wine comes from the abillo grape. Well balanced, clean, crisp, with hints of citrus and a clean aftertaste, this is a wine that can be paired with any cuisine eaten indoors or out.

Fâmega Vinho Verde

You will find this wine, from the cool North Western DOC region of Portugal, to be clean, crisp, and very fresh, with a little tingly sparkle left on your palate. It is very similar to the first pinot grigios imported into the United States from Italy. This exciting young blend of avesso, azul, and pederna' makes it perfect to pair with light cheeses and all types of seafood and salads. Or you can enjoy it just as an aperitif. The alcohol content of Fâmega is 9.5 percent, which makes it the ideal natural, low-calorie white wine.

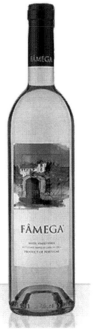

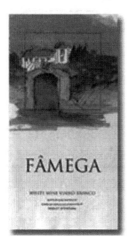

Here are some light wines that may be more familiar.

Kedem (Kosher) Light Wines
Paul Masson Light Chablis

If you intend to buy low-calorie wines, I suggest you purchase only these wines to consume within a few months. These wines are not for cellar storage and therefore may spoil if left on the shelf too long.

Tip for Dieters Watching Their Calories

If you think the sugar in the wine contains all the calories, have I got news for you!

It's the alcohol!

Studies have proven that gram for gram, alcohol has more calories than sugar. You will find that a four-ounce glass of wine will contain about sixty calories. This data doesn't mean you can go out and have wine alone for lunch and still be losing weight. On the contrary, as I said before, wine should be consumed with food while dieting. Remember what the French paradox is all about in an earlier chapter of *Wines for Health*.

Don't leave out the bubbly when choosing a low-calorie sparkler. Look for these prestigious labels with low or no dosage (sugar).

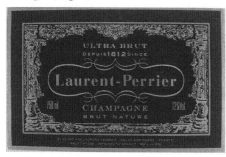

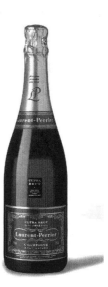

Laurent Perrier "Ultra Brut"

Here is a fine champagne that took off in the 1980s when it was paired with the petite portions of "nouvelle cuisine." Why, you ask? Because "Ultra Brut" was produced with "zero dosage," meaning it has less than three grams of sugar per liter (regular dry or "brut" can contain up to 15 grams per liter).

This very elegant and fresh ABV (alcohol by volume) sparkler makes it a little sharp on your palate. Although the sugar is lacking, it makes a wonderful aperitif. Calories total sixty-five per 4.2-ounce glass.

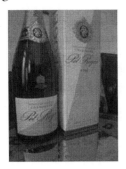

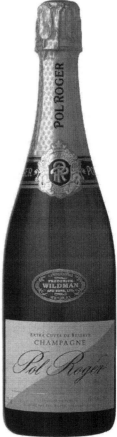

Pol Roger "Pure"

"Pure Brut" from Paul Roger is a pale-colored champagne that is very crisp, clean, and well balanced, a true, exceptional cuvee with no dosage to camouflage it. You can sniff the aromatic flavors of citrus and white floral fragrances in your tulip-shaped glass.

Pure Brut is the perfect accompaniment to all types of seafood or to celebrate any occasion. It is claimed that this champagne was Winston Churchill's favorite bubbly. Only sixty calories per 4.2-

ounce glass and 12 percent ABV, reflecting a no-sugar style.

Ayala "Brut Nature"

This champagne house is owned by the world-renowned Bollinger, specializing in low dosage (lower added-sugar styles). Brut Nature is 12 percent ABV and has no sugar added. Weight watchers will find Brut nature to contain 65 calories per 4.2-ounce glass. Whether it be with sushi or seafood, Brut Nature and its clean, crisp, and citrusy tones will pair well on your palate.

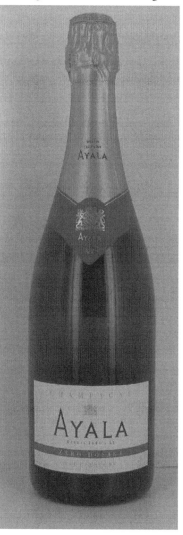

Here is a rough guide to the calories in drinks, which can vary, as they depend on the product and the volume of alcohol. The smallest shot for spirits is 0.84 ounces, and 4.2 ounces is a small glass of wine.

Wine and Champagne (4.5 ounces)

Champagne—95 calories
Sparkling wine— 95 calories
Red wine—85 calories
Rosé—89 calories
Dry white wine—83 calories
Medium white wine—94 calories
Sweet white wine—118 calories

Sherry (0.84 ounces)
Dry sherry—28 calories
Medium sherry— 30 calories
Sweet sherry—35 calories

CHAPTER 13

HEALTHY WINE PAIRING RECIPES

Here are some of my favorite healthy "wine-included recipes."

"The better the wine in your cooking, the better the taste…"

Chateauneuf du Pot Roast with Marinade

Marinade
2 large onions, minced
4 cups of red wine
2 large carrots, minced
3 tablespoons olive oil
1 celery stalk, minced
1 medium onion chopped
3 cups beef stock
2 bay leaves
2 tablespoons tomato paste
1 3-inch strip orange peel

**Combine above ingredients in bowl and blend well.
Add meat, turning to coat all sides. Cover, refrigerate 24
hours.**

1 6-to7- pound beef bottom or top round roast
salt and pepper
1/2 teaspoon dried thyme
1 pound small baking onions, peeled (about32)
1/2 teaspoon dried savory
1/4 teaspoon freshly ground pepper
1 pound rutabaga, peeled and cut into large dice

1/4 cup clarified unsalted butter
1 pound green beans, trimmed and cut into 1-inch pieces

Drain meat, reserving marinade. Pat meat dry. Strain marinade through fine sieve, pressing vegetables on back of spoon to extract liquid; set aside for braising roast. Heat clarified butter in 6-quart Dutch oven or baking dish over medium heat. Add meat, brown all sides, turning with spatula to avoid piercing. Set meat aside. Drain all but 2 tablespoons fat from pan. Return to medium heat. Add minced onions, carrots, and celery and cook until golden brown, 9 to 10 minutes. Add beef stock, tomato paste, salt, pepper, and reserved marinade and bring to simmer. Return meat to pan. Reduce heat to low, cover tightly and simmer gently until meat is barely tender, 2 - 2 1/2 hours.

Stir in diced carrots, baking onions and rutabaga. Cover and cook 15 minutes. Add green beans and continue cooking 20 minutes. Remove from heat, uncover and let cool. Refrigerate at least 1 day, preferably 2 days.

To serve, degrease braising liquid. Place pan over low heat and gently reheat the meat and liquid 1 hour. Slice about 2/3 of the roast and arrange slices with remaining roast on heated platter. Remove vegetables from sauce using slotted spoon and arrange around meat. Taste sauce and reduce to desired concentration of flavor. Spoon some sauce over meat and serve. Serve the remaining sauce separately.

Serve with an Organic Full-Bodied Chateauneuf du Pape, Red Rhone Wine from France.

Stuffed Tacchino Peppers Friulano

6 large green, yellow, red, or orange sweet (bell) peppers
5 tablespoons olive oil
1 large chopped onion
2 cloves garlic (chopped)
2 tablespoons chopped Italian parsley (fresh)
1 pound lean ground turkey (Tacchino)
¼ cup of friulano white wine (Tocai)
Pinch of salt and pepper
¼ cup of grated Locatelli Romano cheese
1 cup cooked rice
1/3 cup pignoli (pine) nuts
16-ounce can Italian crushed tomatoes or marinara sauce
1/4 cup of dry white wine

Use a deep skillet that peppers fit tightly.

Step 1: Cut tops off peppers; discard seeds and membranes. Trim bottoms slightly, if necessary, so peppers can stand up. Set peppers aside.

Step 2: Coat bottom of deep skillet with olive oil. Sauté onions until slightly golden, then add chopped garlic, salt, and pepper. Continue cooking 2 minutes. Then add parsley. Remove mixture from pan and set aside.

Step 3: If needed, slightly coat bottom of skillet again with oil, then add ground turkey and sauté 1-2 minutes.

Step 4: Next add onions, garlic, and wine into turkey mix, stirring frequently. Remove from heat. Add cheese, rice, and pignoli nuts; mix well.

Step 5: Remove all ingredients from skillet and set aside. Pour 8 ounces of tomato sauce into skillet. Stuff all peppers

full with turkey mixture and place in skillet tightly. Pour remaining sauce evenly over each stuffed pepper. Sprinkle additional cheese over each stuffed pepper.

Step 6: Cover skillet and cook over medium heat until peppers are fork tender, approximately 30-45 minutes.

Recipe by Paige Olivia

Grilled Beaujolais Burgers

2 pounds chopped sirloin or chopped buffalo meat
6 shallots, chopped
1/3 cup of grated aged sharp cheddar cheese
1 tablespoon Worcestershire sauce
1 teaspoon garlic powder
¼ cup Beaujolais red wine (French)
Pinch of black pepper
1 tablespoon soy sauce
Lawry's seasoned salt

Step 1: Mix all above ingredients together except Lawry's seasoned salt, then size burgers to your liking.

Step 2: Before grilling burgers, sprinkle lightly with Lawry's seasoned salt.

Step 3: Grill burgers to your taste. Remember, when grilling meat, do not keep turning over. Let the meat cook on one side to seal in the natural juices.

Serve with Louis Jadot Beaujolais Village, France
Recipe by Travis Joseph

Pork Roast Rully

½ cup soy sauce
½ cup of Rully dry white wine (French)
2 cloves of garlic (minced)
1 tablespoon dry mustard
1 teaspoon of ground ginger
1 4-5-pound pork loin roast (boneless)

Step 1: Blend all ingredients except roast.

Step 2: Place roast in plastic bag set in deep bowl.

Step 3: Pour marinade over roast in bag, close, and marinate refrigerate 4 hours.

Step 4: Remove meat and roast at 325 degrees for 2½-3 hours. Discard the   marinade.

Serve with remaining dry white wine Rully, France.
Recipe by Barbara Lee

Chicken Riesling with Grapes
Makes 5 servings.

5 small skinless, boneless chicken breast halves (15 ounces total)
½ cup of German Riesling (medium dry) white wine
(½ teaspoon honey if you can't find very fruity wine)
1 teaspoon of arrowroot
1 teaspoon of instant chicken bouillon granules
1 cup of seedless green or red grapes, halved
Hot whole wheat pasta and herbs to complement chicken

Step 1: Clean and pat dry the chicken. Spray large frying pan

with nonstick coating. **Preheat pan over medium to high heat.**

Step 2: Add chicken and cook about 10 minutes until evenly brown and no longer pink. Remove chicken and keep warm.

Step 3: Mix wine, arrowroot, and bouillon granules and add to the pan. Stir and cook until thick (about 3 minutes) or until you see bubbles.

Step 4: Stir in the grapes until heated and pour over warm chicken. Serve with pasta and herbs.

Serve with a medium dry German wine from the Rhine or Moselle Region.
Recipe by Calysta Brooke

Garlic Shrimp Sauvignon over Risotto

Olive oil
4 cloves of garlic, sliced thin
2 pounds shrimp, deveined and shelled
¼ cup of sauvignon blanc wine (dry)
1 teaspoon Dijon mustard
1 teaspoon Worcestershire sauce
½ teaspoon chili powder
½ teaspoon cayenne pepper (optional)
Chopped parsley
Salt, pepper to taste
1 pound risotto (pasta), prepared according to package directions
Optional: grated Locatelli Romano cheese may be used to complement the dish; sprinkle it on before serving

Step 1: Over medium heat, coat bottom of deep skillet in 2-3 tablespoons olive oil.

Step 2: Add sliced garlic and sauté until lightly brown.

Step 3: Combine all remaining ingredients except risotto in skillet, stirring slowly until shrimp are pink.

Step 4: Strain risotto and pour over shrimp in skillet.

Serve with a Cakebread Cellars Sauvignon Blanc, Napa, California
Recipe by Grayson Michael

Baked Salmon Marsala
Serves 4

Spray olive oil
4 filet salmon steaks—1/3 pound each
Light olive oil
Garlic powder
2 teaspoons parsley (fresh or dried)
Pinch of sea salt
Pepper (optional)
½ cup Marsala wine

Step 1: Use a baking pan in which the salmon steaks will fit tightly (to hold in juices). Spray pan with olive oil lightly.

Step 2: Place salmon steaks on top.

Step 3: Blend olive oil, garlic powder, and parsley in a small bowl. Drizzle over salmon.

Step 4: Sprinkle salt and pepper to taste on salmon.

Step 5: Cover with aluminum foil and bake at 350 degrees approximately 10 minutes. Uncover, pour Marsala over all pieces, and continue to bake, uncovered, an additional 10 minutes.

Serve with an organic Frey white zinfandel (medium dry wine)
Tip: Can be served with creamy white horseradish sauce.
Recipe by Candy Bertuccio

CHAPTER 14
Dedicated to the memory of Marylou Nichols...

SIGN WINES

Just as biodynamic wines are grown compatibly with the earth and go with the lay of the land, moon, and stars; it might be interesting to assign a wine to each sun sign. These recommendations will best suit the palate, as they reflect and complement the personal characteristics of each constellation.

For **Aries** we pick a wine that has accepted the challenge of competition, one that has been recognized in national and international competitions and ranked at the top of its class by wine expert Robert Parker. A winner wants a gold medal for his choice. Give Aries a 2004 Sine Qua Non Poker Face Syrah.

The earthy, hearty, robust Burgundy wines manifest the characteristics of **Taurus**. As no sign would appreciate the Rolls Royce of the wine world more than the sign of the bull, a Louis Jadot Hospice de Beaune Le Montrachet would bring Taurus to the peak of pleasure and reinforce his belief in the power of presents.

Gewurztraminer, tongue-tingling and tongue-tripping, is the wine for **Gemini**. A spicy wine that allows them to enunciate is quite a match for the zodiac's twins. To provide more verbal stimulation, let it wear an Alsatian label that bears the phrases "Reserve Personelle" or "Vendange Tardive" to give them more food for thought.

♋ Sherries and ports that can be used for cooking as well as desserts are "faves" for **Cancer**. Some are packaged in heart-shaped bottles that also make for beautiful additions to this sign's collector's items.

♌ **Leo** will pick a traditional, historic wine of noble heritage. One that is well respected and enhances their image would add an even finer touch. That can only be a Pauillac or Pomerol from Bordeaux with the name "Baron Philippe de Rothschild" on the label.

♍ A perfect pick for **Virgo** is a wine that has earned a flawless reputation and lives up to even the most critical palate. That is Chateau Mouton Rothschild 1982. One of the best vintages of the last century, it is also working for you when it is sleeping in your cellar.

♎ **Libra** will enjoy a wine that is "in" and the height of good taste (no pun intended). To appeal to Libra's artistic eye, it will be contained in a beautiful bottle with a stylish label. This sign's choice would be Mionetto Cartizze.

♏ In tune with the regenerative power of **Scorpio** is a wine that has been so greatly transformed that there is barely a trace of the old left. Austria's new-style Gruner Veltliner has always had the potential for great things and has come back renewed and refreshed to become one of the most popular wines today.

A wine from a land far away will set the stage for *Sagittarius* and give him a sense of freedom and adventure. How much farther away can he get than Australia, whose wines are all "quietly sensational"? While imagining himself as Crocodile Dundee, he can add a bit of reality to his own vision by sipping a reserve Shiraz like Hardy Tintara.

A "power wine" noted for its reputation and rank in the world is the *Capricorn* choice. Coming from a prestigious company, it must be recognized for quality and value and ready to stand alone as a good investment. Chateau Lafite Rothschild, a wine of wealth and position, would meet all the requirements of this upwardly mobile sign.

In this new age of *Aquarius* there are many up-and-coming wines to be paired with today's cross-cultured cuisine. One of the up-and-coming eco-organic wines mentioned in this book can be tried with a sure-fire result of satisfaction.

An excellent pick for *Pisces*, a Neptune-ruled planet, is a wine that will go well with seafood. That is an Italian

Friulano wine (formerly Tocai). A dreamy wine, it can also be used in the simple recipe above for peppers stuffed with lean ground turkey (Stuffed Tachino Peppers Friulano).

A Votre Santé—To Your Health

For Your Info…

Now that I have raised your eyebrows to the health benefits of wine. It might take a few years before the FDA grants full approval for resveratrol supplements. Before the FDA grants approval, an optical therapeutic dosage and clinical studies have to be established. If you base it on animal studies, a safe dosage would be around 500 milligrams a day.

In March 2009, *60 Minutes* interviewed Dr. Christoph Westphal and Harvard biochemist David Sinclair. These men have been researching resveratrol using laboratory mice and claim it delays the aging process and prevents many gerontological diseases.

These men have invented a resveratrol pill which is equivalent to drinking one hundred glasses of wine (without a hangover). David Sinclair said the pill should be available by 2015. There are, however, resveratrol pills selling now, but most are mixed with other supplements, and the dosage is far less than the Harvard duo's new pill.

Loss of My Wine Friend

The year was 1985 and I had just produced the first television show on wine in the United States. The show was broadcast in seventeen major cities on cable television. I was thirty-eight years old with a dream to teach people about wine, which at that time I couldn't do on regular television.

I can't tell you how excited I was when Marci Mondavi answered my letter inviting her dad, Robert Mondavi, on my show. Wow, I got California's godfather of wine as a guest.

The studio was way out in Suffolk County, Long Island, at least one hour's drive from New York City, where Robert always visited. I knew I had to do some fast scheduling to interview him in the city. But where? No one had ever heard of my show, and I couldn't afford to rent a studio. I had an idea to interview him in a prestigious restaurant, but because of preparation before lunch and dinner, the times were not accommodating. I decided to call the Hotel Pierre and ask to use its restaurant. When the management heard I was interviewing Robert Mondavi, they were gracious enough to give me a large suite for my taping.

I remember that day very clearly. I was so nervous because Robert, who said to call him Bob, was my first wine celebrity guest. The segment was to take ten to fifteen minutes and, according to the director, break for a commercial. The producers had two Victorian chairs set up facing each other in front of a beautiful mantel and fireplace. Cue cards were ready, and then Marci walk in with her dad and introductions were made. Ten minutes before we sat down, while they were putting the microphones on us, Bob asked me about the show and said how impressed he was that I was following my dream to teach people about wine and the fine families behind the labels—"good families like yours and mine." At that time, the press was bashing drinking in any way, regardless of whether it was hard liquor, beer, or wine. Good wine was getting a bad rap because reports of some driving-while-impaired accidents involving young adults said wine was the cause. But, the press forgot to mention it was wine coolers and over indulgence.

I guess Bob knew I was a bit nervous, and after our brief talk, he made me feel like I was talking to my own grandfather.

We sat down for the interview on camera. I was much more relaxed while sharing a couple of glasses of his cabernet sauvignon reserve, and an interview that was to last fifteen minutes could have turned into enough taping for an hour-long show.

Bob told my audience that he was on a mission, and that mission was to enjoy the finer wines, and that wine is to enjoy and have fun with as long as we drink in moderation. We know that too much of one thing is not good for you. But as long as we enjoy that one thing in moderation, it will be fine.

I was honored to meet with Bob a year later on Long Island at the Garden City Hotel's Georgio Restaurant. Bob was on a new mission pairing his wines with dishes prepared by top chefs worldwide. Sound familiar? Drinking in moderation and pairing wines with fine cuisine.

Just to think I was part of sharing his dreams with thousands of people on my television and radio shows, through my wine etiquette lectures and the books I have written, is gratifying.

Here was a man I admired because he followed his dream as a wine crusader-pioneer. His wines speak for his entire family, who follows his dream and puts quality first in every bottle it produces.

My heart goes out to the Mondavi family for its loss of Robert Mondavi. I know the Bertuccio family will never forget him.

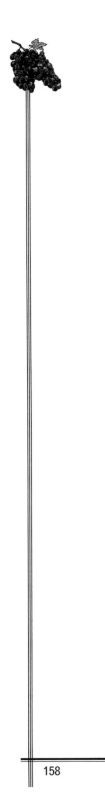

REFERENCES

1. *Wine and Health by Indage April 10, 2003*
   www.indianwine.com/winenowebpage.htm

2. *Wine and Health Issues. April 7, 2003*
   (www.delhiwineclub.com/winehealth.htm).

3. *BBC News, September 19, 2000 Red Wine "can stop herpes"*
   http://news.bbc.co.uk/1/health/931850.stm

4. *Wine and Health Issues. April 7, 2003 Wine and Cold Research*
   (www.delhiwineclub.com/winehealth.htm).

5. *Reuters Health, New York. Source: American Journal of Epidemiology 2002;*
   155:332-338

6. *Sources: LiveScience, Reuters, HealthDay News*

7. *Wikipedia.org 2008 Benefits of Armagnac*

8. *Bell D. S. Alcohol and the NIDDM patient, .Diabetes Care 1996 May ; Al Qatari, M., M. F. Smith, and P. V. Taberner. Chronic ethanol consumption ameliorates the maturity-onset-diabetes-obesity syndrome in CBA mice, Alcohol January 31, 1996*

9. *Antiagingbydesign.com/Harvard Medical School Study*

10. *Elizabeth Holmgren, Dir. Dept. of Research At the Wine Institute.*
    Beekmanwine.com

11. *Wine and health. - 26th March 2006 at 4Hoteliers,*
www.4hoteliers.com/4hots_fshw.php?mwi=1231

12. *Wine and Health by Indage*
(www.aidaindia.org/aida/Wine_Health.htm)

13. *Drink and Keep diabetes at bay*
(www.aidaindia.org/aida/drink.htm

14. *Harvard Medical Study - Fri. 27 March 2009*
reduxatrol.com

15. *Evan H. Siemann and Creasy, "Concentration of the Phytoalexin Resveratrol in Wine,"*
www.news.cornell.edu/chronicle/98/2.5.98/resveratrol.html

16. *Resveratrol may help treat fatty liver. Colihan, Kelly. Web MD Health News. October 15, 2008. Reviewed by Louise Chang, MD.*

17. *Light Drinking May Help Keep Leg Arteries Clear NEW YORK (Reuters Health) SOURCE: American Journal of Epidemiology 2002;155:332-338.*

18. *Fountain of Youth, Colihan, Kelly. Web MD Health News. October 15, 2008. Reviewed by Louise Chang, MD*

19. *Alcohol benefits in wine, Colihan, Kelly. Web MD Health News. October 15, 2008. Reviewed by Louise Chang, MD, health benefits of wine*

Official recommendation in the 1995 *Dietary Guidelines for Americans, Fourth Edition*, published by the U.S. Food and Drug Administration.

AUTHOR'S BIO...

For the past four decades, oenologist, author, wine writer, and radio/television show host Joseph Bertuccio has been involved in all phases of the wine industry, from the planting of organic vine stocks to consulting for the State Department on a dinner wine for the President of the United States. Joseph has also consulted for Harvard University's International Affairs Department on wine etiquette and wine selection for prestigious dinners and seminars for members of the United Nations Security Council, ambassadors to the United Nations, former Secretary of State Madeleine Albright, and former Permanent Ambassador of the Russian Federation and present Foreign Minister Sergey Lavaroff.

Joseph has been a guest on ABC's *Regis and Kathy Lee*, the Food Network's *Hot Off the Grill* with Bobby Flay, and New York's Metro Channel *Health Show* with Mary Mucci. He is scheduled for continuing appearances on several national talk shows and has hosted his own show, *That's the Spirit*, on national cable TV.

Joseph's first book, *Join Me in the Wine World*, was an instant success that led him to publish two additional editions. It is still very popular among many wine novices.

Joseph's current book, *Wines for Health*, takes the savvy reader into a world of healthy wine drinking that will cure the body of many ailments. Joseph delves into many wine categories, such as biodynamic wines, organic wine, vegetarian wines, vegan wines, and nonalcoholic wines. *Wines for Health* is a mini-course in "healthy wine-know." With a simple and spelled-out approach, it takes you directly to intelligent and satisfying wine choices.

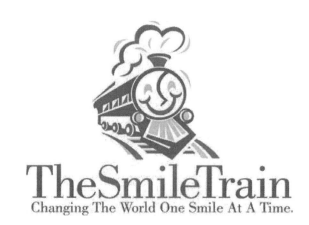

TheSmileTrain
Changing The World One Smile At A Time.

A percentage of proceeds from the book are donated to the Smile Train, Changing the World One Smile at a Time. The Smile Train empowers local surgeons around the world to provide life-changing cleft palate surgery. It gives desperate children not just a new smile—but a new life. Learn more at http://www.smiletrain.org/.

Quick Reference Guide

__ACIDOSIS__ — excessive acid in the body fluids.

__ALZHEIMER'S DISEASE__ — a brain disorder that is similar to dementia. It is characterized by memory loss and severe behavioral changes and has no current cure.

__ATHEROSCLEROSIS__ — A building up of plaque in the artery walls. This can be controlled by watching what one is eating. Exercise is also good to combat this problem.

__AUTOIMMUNE DISEASE__ — a case of mistaken identity, when the body begins attacking its own healthy tissue. Autoimmune conditions include rheumatoid arthritis and lupus.

__CATARACTS__ — the clouding of the lens in an eye. The lens works to focus the light to the retina, and with cataracts, the light is partially blocked, much like a smudge on a camera lens.

__CHOLERA BACTERIA__ — a severe infection caused by the bacterium Vibrio cholerae, which primarily affects the small intestine. The main symptoms include profuse watery diarrhea and vomiting.

__CHOLESTEROL__ — a fatty-looking substance that is found in your bloodstream; too much of it can cause heart problems, like a heart attack or even a stroke.

COLORECTAL POLYP — a growth that sticks out of the lining of the colon or rectum.

CORONARY HEART DISEASE (CHD) — is narrowing of the small blood vessels that supply blood and oxygen to the heart.

CYTOKINES — enzymes and proteins produced by the cells of the immune system. Their main purpose is as regulators during the generation of an immune response to the detection of a foreign body or substance.

DEMENTIA — change in your brain function. Asking the same question over and over, not being able to follow directions, and getting confused easily are signs of dementia. Dementia can be caused by Alzheimer's disease.

DUODENUM — the first part of the small intestine. It is located between the stomach and the middle part of the small intestine, or jejunum. After foods mix with stomach acid, they move into the duodenum, where they mix with bile from the gallbladder and digestive juices from the pancreas.Absorption of vitamins, minerals, and other nutrients begins in the duodenum.

DYSREGULATION — a state of stress, being overwhelmed, or pain that is out of one's ability to tolerate. Negative behaviors arise from this state. The absolute fundamental cause of dysregulation is fear.

E CPU BACTERIA — *Escherichia coli* is a member of the coliform group. Coliform is a bacteria found in fecal matter of warm-blooded animals. Foods and water are often tested for the coliform bacteria level.

ENDOMETRIAL CANCER — cancer of the uterine lining. Of course, this only occurs in women, as men do not have a uterus. It is treatable if it is caught in its early stages.

FERMENTATION — the process by which cells release energy under anaerobic conditions (generally). Major products of fermentation are ethanol, lactic acid, and hydrogen gas. Fermentation of sugars by yeast is typically used as the source of ethanol for alcoholic beverages.

FLAVONOIDS — also called vitamin P and citrin. They are helpful in prevention of cancers and are antioxidants. They are found in citrus fruits, dark chocolates, wine, and teas.

FREE RADICALS — atoms, ions, or molecules with unpaired electrons. They have an open shell configuration. Free radicals are highly reactive. They have important roles in many chemical processes, including within the human body. They've even been implicated in the process of aging! Organic free radicals were discovered in 1900 by Moses Gomberg.

GASTROENTEROLOGY — the study of the entire gastrointestinal tract, including the esophagus, stomach, intestines, anus, liver, gallbladder, etc.

GASTRONOMY — of the study of the relationships between food and culture. The word also often refers to the artwork of cooking.

HERPES SIMPLEX — an infection that mainly affects the mouth or genital area.

HDL — high density lipoprotein, a form of "good" cholesterol. Lipoproteins are proteins in the blood that move cholesterol, triglycerides, and other lipids to various tissues.

HYPOGLYCEMIA — a condition that occurs when your blood sugar (glucose) is too low.

LDL — low-density lipoprotein in your blood. LDL is a type of cholesterol. Too much LDL in the blood can clog arteries.

LEES — sediment settling during fermentation, especially in wine; dregs.

LYMPHOCYTE — any of the nearly colorless cells found in the blood, lymph, and lymphoid tissues, constituting approximately 25 percent of white blood cells and including B cells, which function in humoral immunity (protects against free-floating foreign molecules (antigens), and T cells, which function in cellular immunity (bind to the surface of other cells that display the antigen and trigger a response.

MELONOMA — a type of cancer that is found in the pigment-producing cells on the skin (meianocytes). When meianocytes go crazy and overgrow, the growth is called a melanoma, and it needs to be removed before it spreads.

MICROCLIMATE — a small region within a greater region, where the climate within the small region is unique and differs from the bigger region.

MITOCHONDRIA — the main part of the cell. This is really the area that makes the energy that the cell can use to help the body with its breathing function.

OBESITY — body weight that is much greater than what is considered healthy.

OBGYN — obstetrics and gynecology. Obstetric and gynecologic surgery refers to procedures that are performed to treat a variety of conditions affecting the female.

ORGANELLAS — small organs. A cell has nine different parts that makes it work, and each of these is in organelles. Some of the parts in a cell are the nucleus, cell membrane, and cytoplasm.

PEPTIC ULCERS — erosions in the lining of the stomach or duodenum (the first part of the small intestine).

PERIODONTAL DISEASE — disease affecting the gums, which consist of the gingiva, periodontal ligament, cementum, and alveolar bone.

PROPHYLACTIC — a preventive measure. The word comes from the Greek for "an advance guard," an apt term for a measure taken to fend off a disease or another unwanted consequence. A prophylactic is a medication or a treatment designed and used to prevent a disease from occurring.

PULMONARY DISEASE — any disease of the lungs or respiratory system. The term can include diseases of the pulmonary artery or vein as well as of the lungs. The most common pulmonary disease is COPD, which stands for chronic obstructive pulmonary disease. RESVERATROL — a natural compound found in grapes, mulberries, peanuts, and other plants or food products, especially red wine, that may protect against cancer and cardiovascular disease by acting as an antioxidant, antimutagen, and anti-inflammatory.

STREPTOCOCCUS MUTANS — a bacteria commonly found in the human oral cavity and a significant contributor to tooth decay.

TANNIN — a bitter plant polyphenol. It plays a major part in the processes of ripening fruit and aging wine; it's the modification or declining level of tannin that changes the flavors. Tannin is what causes that puckering sensation you get in your mouth after you've tasted unripened fruit or red wine.

TEETOTALER — one who practices or advocates abstinence from all alcoholic beverages.

TERROIR — originally a French term used about wine, coffee, and tea to denote the special characteristics that geography bestowed upon these beverages.

TYPHOID FEVER — a bacterial infection characterized by diarrhea, systemic disease, and a rash; most commonly caused by the bacteria *Salmonella typhi*.

VITICULTURIST — a professional whose business is grapes. Viticulturists play important roles in the production of wine. These individuals usually strive to ensure that the grapes that will be used are grown in a manner that will provide maximum yield and flavor. Some trained viticulturists, however, work in other areas of the wine industry as well.

VINOTHEREPY — a beauty therapy process where the residue of wine making (the pips and pulp) are rubbed into the skin. The pulp is said to have excellent exfoliating qualities and help reduce the problems associated with aging. Vinotherapy is becoming popular in holiday resorts in Spain, Portugal, and France, where visitors are offered spa treatments, including vinotherapy.

Index

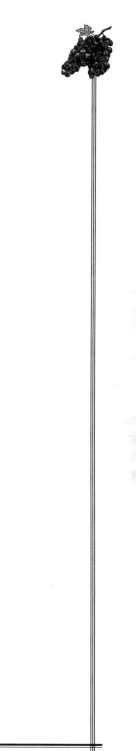